TAKE B YOUR YOUR OUTSIDE MINDSET

LIVE LONGER, PREVENT DEMENTIA, AND CONTROL YOUR CHRONIC ILLNESS

Verla Fortier

TAKE BACK YOUR OUTSIDE MINDSET: LIVE LONGER, PREVENT DEMENTIA, AND CONTROL YOUR CHRONIC ILLNESS

COVER DESIGN BY JANE DIXON
INTERIOR DESIGN BY VANYA DRUMCHIYSKA

ISBN: 978-1-69076-675-9

～　FOR MY FAMILY　∽

CONTENTS

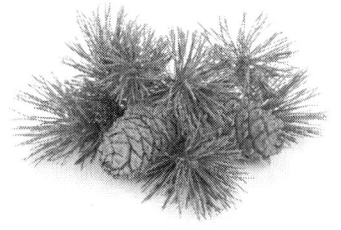

INTRODUCTION

The atmosphere around trees may be the most powerful natural medicine we have access to, yet most of us are completely unaware of it.

> —Diana Beresford-Kroeger, a 35-year-long career as a botanist, author, lecturer, and medical researcher in the fields of botany, medical biochemistry, organic chemistry, and nuclear chemistry

A mindset is a belief that orients the way we handle situations— the way we sort out what is going on in our lives and what we should do about it.

> —Ellen Langer, PhD, social psychologist at Harvard University, 40 year career as researcher and author in the science of mindlessness and mindfulness

Imagine a Miracle Drug

Imagine a universal medication that has no side effects and is available to anyone who needs it. This same drug is proven to improve short- and long-term memory, increase your ability to concentrate, and help you to problem solve. This medication not only helps you keep track of things and remember the steps in the task at hand, it lifts your mood, boosts your energy level, and gives you self-confidence. To top it off, this miracle drug costs you nothing.

That's the dramatic promise of time spent outside, near trees and in urban green space.

My Lupus Story

When serious systemic lupus hit me in my 60's, I was worried about dying too early, about losing my mind to dementia and rampant chronic illness.

I tried meditating, but it proved too much work. I tried manufacturing positive thinking, which was even more exhausting.

I did what felt best to me. I stayed inside like everyone else who is sick. I stayed inside because my dermatologist told me to avoid the sun. I stayed inside because I felt terrible. I stayed inside because I wanted to figure out what was going on and get a handle on how to crawl out of this dark hole.

Instead of finding a way out, I was paralyzed by profound losses that just kept coming—my father had died of complications caused by multiple sclerosis and my mother of dementia.

I knew too well the long process of deterioration to death.

My Experience as a Healthcare Professional

As a nurse, researcher, professor, and administrator I knew about chronic disease. I knew how lupus could take down every organ in my body. I cared for patients as they died from lupus. As a healthcare team, we did everything we could, but the disease would keep firm hold of the whole body until the very end.

Most of us know that chronic diseases, also known as life-time conditions, cannot be cured. And we know that nearly half of Canadians (44%) and Americans (45%) have at least one chronic disease.

My first thought after my diagnosis was that each additional chronic illness shaves years off of a person's life.

Medical Solutions Not Enough

I also knew the reality of day to day medical work. There is little time to research something new. And there is huge pressure on the medical health system to provide all the answers.

The science of medicine has gained powerful tools like pharmacology and diagnostic tests. Medical science is the basis of evidence-based patient care.

This science drives medical guidelines and protocols for patient care. As nurses and doctors, we are off to the races with our shared assessment and treatment options. Doctors have roughly 15 minutes per patient visit to get everything covered.

When I suddenly became the patient, these medical solutions were not enough. I put my health in the hands of many physician specialists, but none of this worked. My fears only multiplied.

Sharp Left Turn

Although I spent my career in healthcare, I took a sharp left turn into tree research. It was both uncomfortable and exhilarating. It was hard to find the research, scary to go after it, and even more terrifying to actually write about it.

But I did the work anyway. And I had no idea where the research was going. I just followed my fears. Now I believe the truth of it in my heart.

The Striking Findings

The striking findings about trees, green space, living longer, preventing dementia, and controlling chronic disease is there. It was hard to find and pull together. But it is brilliant. The research is so good it cannot be ignored.

This research is a powerful interdisciplinary soup. It is not in one type of science. It is in the fields of geometry, mathematics, physics, health geography, economics, environmental neuroscience, psychology, biology, botany, and forestry medicine.

All the things we fear losing most in the aging process—our lives, memory, energy, focus, health, and happiness—are boosted by spending time outside. And there is solid research to prove it.

In this book, I did not dumb down the research, but attempted to present each study's methodology in "how they did it" sections so you can be empowered by it too. And then, as Harvard social psychologist Ellen Langer says, "what the mind believes, the body delivers." Once you have the knowledge and act on it, your body will change.

Why I Wrote This Book

At first, I wrote this book for me. I needed it to get better. And it worked. Now I want to get this information into the hands of my demographic. I want you to understand and believe the specifics of this green space research. I want you to feel the relief, exuberance, and new hope, that I now have.

In this book, I share the feelings and emotions driven by my journey of loss and discovery. When I learned I had lupus, I had so many fears I could not articulate them. I wrote this book because at my core I was terrified. I knew the limited world of medical care. I knew the disease.

Before my diagnosis it was so easy to be distracted by other things. But when you have a serious diagnosis it is gut wrenching. And the clock is ticking. I asked myself, "Is this the way I want to spend the rest of my life?"

I Wish

I often wish that during those dark days I had had access to a book that articulated not only how I felt, but also showed me what no one else in the aging and chronic care community was talking about: the power of green space on our specific worries.

Aging with chronic disease is my demographic. We have the most to gain by using this research.

I wish I had known that spending time close to trees— something that required no effort, treatment that I did not have to buy—would have such a profound effect on my mental and physical health.

Mindset Is Often Overlooked

Yes, my body was breaking down, but I wish I had considered my mindset as well. A large part of aging and chronic disease is wrapped up in a silent mindset of fear and self-doubt. We don't address it, but we should as it shapes much of our world view.

This Research Will Change Your Life

Rather than having you look for it on your own, I want to help you discover this outside research through my story. I want to save you time and money and help you to feel better than ever. I want you to know how to live longer, stress less, and prevent dementia. I want the research to take you to a new place. In your green space you will be relaxed and in control of your life with chronic disease.

In this short book, I share my journey and the outside research information that changed my life.

If you have limited energy, time, and money, an unsettled mind, and are in pain, this little book will show you how you can dramatically change your mind and body as you age with or without chronic disease.

Overview of This Book

Part 1: A Bad Feeling

Even the constant rollercoaster that life throws us into may not force us to consider changing our mindset. In this first part, I share my divorce story before I was diagnosed with lupus. I was too busy and then too sick to go outside very often. I never really thought about it.

I fully realize that nothing can prepare you for a shattering, progressive chronic disease diagnosis. My own life is a great example of how messy things can get when you are in your sixties and told you have chronic diseases. I share my losses, how I began to think after I heard the news, and my reasons for hiding inside.

Part 2: The Effect of Green Space on Worry, Life Span, Memory, Attention, Brain Structure, Motivation, and Effort

Part two of this book gets into the science of how green space affects your health. The research results are as wide as the title of this book promises.

For example, Professor Greg Bratman, a biologist in Environment and Forest Sciences at the University of Washington, showed that being near trees and green space for 90 minutes every day changes our thinking from negative to positive. And then his team showed that green space "improves cognition." Cognition, in their study, referred to short- and long-term memory, ability to concentrate and to learn new things.

Marc Berman, Engineer and Professor of Psychology at the University of Chicago, showed that being in green space restores your ability to pay attention.

Professor Richard Mitchell, an epidemiologist and geographer at the University of Glasgow, conducted a study that showed how in less than 5 minutes spent outside near green space, your mood and self-esteem do get a boost.

Professor Richard Taylor, a physicist in the Departments of Physics and Psychology at the University of Oregon, showed that by looking into the branches of a tree you will decrease your stress levels by 60%.

Professor Ellen Langer, a social psychologist at Harvard University, shows in her forty years of research how to be present without meditating. Now in her seventies, she sums up her work by saying that "our beliefs are the only things that matter."

Part 3: Ways of Being Outside

By this point, you probably think that you need to camp out in the woods for best results—but that is not really the case. In part three, I focus on the scientific research that presents the ways you can benefit from the outdoors.

The scientists I mention treat time spent near trees and green space as "dosages." And the benefits are treated as "response." Think of your green space as your new pharmacy.

I give you ways to jumpstart your success with:

— Tree time "dosages" and locations as tested by researchers;

— Ways of noticing while you are outside;

— Words that work when you are outside;

— 100+ outdoor practices to create and keep your outside mindset.

By the end of this book, you will have your own outside mindset and you will know exactly how to live longer, prevent dementia, and control your chronic illness. As a result, you will be calm and confident. You will be able to keep track of things and figure out problems. You will take back control of your life—with or without chronic disease. It will be dramatically easy. It will be effortless. It will be fun and freeing.

PART 1:
A BAD FEELING

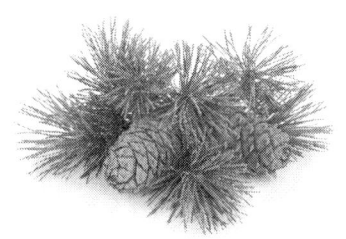

CHAPTER 1:
MINDSET IS DIFFERENT WHEN YOU ARE YOUNG

Even if we live in a way that keeps us unaware of our mindset, we do have one. Our mindset is a mental tool that helps us make sense of things. It is our framework for moving forward (or backward).

Until I knew I had a chronic disease, I never considered my mindset. My solution to the roller coaster of life was simple. I kept the kids as my main priority, earned more income, and headed to the gym whenever possible.

I had several jobs and no time to think. This scenario worked for me.

Chronic Disease Diagnosis

When, at the age of 63, I learned I had systemic lupus, I felt immobilized and hid inside my house.

I wish I had known that although my body was acting strange, I had not lost control over my mind. I wish I had known I could have had agency over my thoughts and emotions.

After My Divorce

When my ex-husband and I divorced, I was left to take care of my two small boys at home. Looking into their expectant and confused eyes, it was clear to me that I needed to bounce back. And I did. *We* did.

I revved up my income by supplementing my hospital administration position. I became an Assistant Professor at McMaster University School of Nursing. I took on a full teaching course load.

At the time, I did not need to consider the thought/emotion connection to my new single mother situation.

I knew how to avoid that unproductive mental chatter. I knew how to avoid my thoughts. I switched the channel to work, loving my kids, regular gym workouts, and binge eating.

Rewriting the Script

After the divorce settled, our world did come crashing down. And yet I was able to rewrite the script very early on.

A work colleague said he was sorry to hear about the divorce. Without thinking I responded, "It was his idea—but it was a good one."

We laughed. And to me this became the truth.

My divorce story.

Held Hostage

If only I had been able to hold on to that mindset. However, I did not learn to let go of my divorce. For years I held on to regrets and bitterness. My inner voice worked overtime with all the "what ifs" and "if onlys." I understand now that this is normal for a period of time, but these thoughts persisted for 15 years.

At no time did I stop and ask myself, "Are these thoughts helping me feel better? Will their recurrence improve my life?" I was unable to move on.

It was not until my chronic illness diagnosis, a decade and a half later, that I found the name for this constant rehashing. I stumbled upon it when I was researching the health benefits of trees. My thought pattern fell into the category of "negative rumination."

I was, as award-winning, 70-something Harvard psychologist Ellen Langer says, "knee deep in regret, resentment, and mindlessness."

Unaware

Until two years ago, well into my 60's, I did not know I had a chronic disease. It turned out, after a series of tests, that I have systemic lupus.

Two years ago, before I heard my diagnosis, I lived in Burlington, Ontario, Canada. This was home to my two boys and me. We lived in a huge, modern, suburban "mansion," as we first called it when we moved in.

After the divorce, I wanted to keep our family home for the boys—as a symbol of our stability. It was our refuge. We loved our home, our neighbours, and our community—a lot.

Working More Than Ever

The mansion, however, came with a big mortgage which required me to work more. This was fine with me. I was completely engaged in my career. My university teaching role enhanced my hospital administration position. The healthcare research in both positions drew me in.

Roughly 10 years later, I hated getting in my car and driving to work. I found it painful to sit in meetings. My legs cramped and sometimes seized, but I considered these symptoms a normal part of the aging process.

Still I worked on research proposals in my office late into the evenings. The muscle and bone pain became so severe I often struggled to walk back to my car at the end of the work day. I was glad none of my colleagues saw me hobble to my car.

I Loved Going to the Gym

Despite everything, or because of it, I dedicated my time after work to the Goodlife gym. Very often my crampy legs refused to climb the stairs on their own, and I had to hang on to the railings to keep going up.

Once I entered my safe haven, I would start moving right away which helped me feel better. The gym was my lifeline at that time. I had a close girlfriend who was my workout buddy there. We did all the classes together and kept each other sane.

Later, when I finally made it home, I would eat everything in sight. I ate myself into a stupor and fell into bed.

The kids helped themselves to leftovers of whatever I had managed to cook on the weekends. During the week they were looking after themselves. We were in survival mode.

Every morning I wanted to drive by my highway work exit and end up anywhere else but there.

I did not know I had an illness. I had worries, sure, but so did everybody else. My problems were nothing special.

When a rash appeared on my face, my GP referred me to a dermatologist who burned it off, dismissing the rash as a "sunspot."

This only made it worse. I purchased cosmetic products to try to conceal the spreading red rash on my face. I carried on with my busy life—smiling more and hoping no one would notice.

~Questions

When you were younger and things happened that you did not like, how did you cope?

What worked? What did not?

CHAPTER 2:
GETTING A DIAGNOSIS

The moment the second dermatologist looked at me I knew she saw something. She examined every red rash and bald patch on my scalp. She did this with care. Then she reached for my hands. Her voice softened.

Oh no. I had a bad feeling about this.

She said that all my clinical symptoms indicated lupus. "We will do a biopsy and draw blood to see if it is the skin type or the system type."

The bloodwork revealed my condition as systemic lupus. This is the serious type which usually means high risk of organ involvement. The kidneys, heart, lungs, and liver are most susceptible.

There are blood tests to diagnose lupus. They are: Antinuclear antibodies and DNA-Binding antibodies. These, combined with clinical symptoms, produce a diagnosis. I had both. This showed "exacerbation of the disease." My condition was active.

Getting this diagnosis was like striking a match. Once struck, the match does not light again.

There was no going back.

A Progressive Disease That Has No Cure

The words of my doctor seared into my mind. "This is a progressive chronic disease that has no cure. Medications can help control the symptoms. We need to start you on the medication Plaquenil for the face rash and hair loss. This might help the joint, muscle, and nerve pain. Avoid sunlight; it can damage your DNA."

I did not expect any psychological counselling beyond her kindness. The visit was over. Physical symptom control was the priority. I got it.

How long will I live? I thought to myself, but in my stunned state, I could not verbalize this question to my physician. I was a nursing professor so I knew I could answer my own questions. As soon as I got home, I began my research. I googled: "Peer reviewed clinical trials on life expectancy with chronic disease."

In an instant, I had my answer:

"Life expectancy decreases by approximately 1.8 years with each chronic condition."

Ok, I could live with that. But what about systemic lupus? I had lost many patients to lupus over the years. "Multi-organ failure" sealed the lupus fate.

Is My Chronic Disease Different?

I narrowed my search criteria. I wanted to know about life expectancy of women who suffered from systemic lupus. Next I googled, "Peer reviewed clinical trials on life expectancy for women with systemic lupus."

This headline hit hard:

"Lupus Patients, Especially Women, Die at Younger Ages."

Stanford University published the study in 2017. The results showed that "women with systemic lupus erythematosus (SLE) in the U.S. live on average 22 years less—and men an average of 12 fewer years—than members of the same sex among the public at large."

At 65, I felt like my time was up.

I Was an Insider: I Knew the Answers

As a nurse with a Master's in Health Sciences I was an insider. I knew the limited world of medical care. Medications, blood tests, diagnostic tests, trying one thing and then another. I worried. I knew how we, in the healthcare system, categorized disease and locked into treatment options.

This I knew from experience: there weren't many tools in the medical system box: Diagnostic tests to confirm the diagnosis. Medication to control the symptoms.

The healthcare team follows shared Medical Clinical Practice Guidelines and treatment protocols. Then they follow a treatment trial-and-error process combined with medical procedures. Caring is always a part of the process. But there is never enough time.

My Brain Was Wired for Hopelessness

I knew not to expect emotional support from the healthcare system. My brain was already wired for hopelessness. My past failures resurfaced, and my emotions took over.

My father had died of complications of multiple sclerosis and my mother of dementia. My brain knew about long chronic illness deterioration until death. It wasn't beyond the ordinary that my emotions went there, taking my past failures along.

I felt doomed and did not even stop to question the truth of that feeling.

My Go-To Option of Working Harder Was Gone

In the past years, my consistent strategy for handling stressful events had been to dig deep and find the grit to work harder. Just add another job to the mix.

But when chronic illness came along, my go-to option was not there.

I did not have the energy to work harder and that led to feelings of worthlessness and loss of self-esteem.

Shame did not delay. My emotions struck harder than before.

∼Questions

Have you or a loved one received a diagnosis where you felt devastated?

What were your first thoughts?

Chapter 3: Shattered

No one else in my life had lupus. Not my work colleagues, not my friends, not my family.

I thought there must be some mistake. I was so healthy—how had this happened? And how would it affect my career, my income, my freedom, my body, my brain?

Overnight I lost my status as a healthy professional.

What about money? I still had one son in an expensive university on the other side of the country.

The losses felt so vast I could not keep track of them. How could I possibly find solutions to all these issues?

Looking forward, all I could see was thick fog that seemed to engulf everything in my world.

Looking backward, I saw everything lupus had taken from me. Shattered, I felt everything this disease had forced me to relinquish.

Negative Thought Circles

My negative thoughts sunk in circles that didn't help. I kept thinking:

I can't do this.

I feel terrible.

I am too old for this.
Why is my body not like everyone else's body?
Why is my body going haywire?
I should be able to figure out why.
If only I was not so screwed.
I should be able to cope.

No Longer Equal

I no longer felt like I was an equal as I discouraged family and friends from visiting.

Activities of daily living became a chore. Taking a shower took enormous energy. I had a hard time cleaning up the kitchen. Cooking for myself was out of the question.

I tried to figure out what might come next.

As soon as I mastered one symptom, another appeared.

~*Questions*

Did you rehash thoughts about you and your illness?
Did you share these thoughts with anyone close to you?

CHAPTER 4:
WHO AM I NOW?

Who was I now anyway? My self-image was shattered. Every day a new loss dawned on me.

I was too ashamed to share these with anyone.

The biggest threat to my sanity was fear. I was afraid of death, fatigue, pain, more disfiguring hair loss, and facial rashes.

In my life before the lupus diagnosis I had valued how I looked, moved, and laughed. But these were gone now.

I knew about the famous stages of grief and how they don't have to happen in sequence. But mine seemed to have no resolution.

My anxiety reoccurred in many ways and would lash at me over and over again. I knew the consequences were becoming severe. Still I did not want to share my problem with anyone, not even family or friends.

I kept adding to the total sum of my losses. They were enormous. And repetitive.

My body image, once a strength, fractured. I was no longer good-looking, sexy, or healthy.

I kept looking backwards to who I had been and comparing my past self to the person I thought I had turned into.

So Many Reasons to Stay Inside

Looking good had always mattered to me. I had relied on it.

Lupus causes severe inflammation in the body, and hair often becomes a casualty. The face and scalp become the usual targets of skin inflammation related to this disease.

Hair Loss

I was losing hair from the top of my head. I kept finding more and more bald patches as new clumps kept falling out. And I was losing my eyebrows. "Scarring alopecia" is a lupus symptom. The hair follicles become scarred, and hair cannot grow back in those places.

I had never considered exactly how much self-esteem I had invested in my hair.

Body Rashes

Things didn't stop there. The lupus telltale "butterfly"-shaped rash soon appeared across my face. I also had ruby-red, itchy, painful slashes on my neck, chest, arms, ears, and forehead. I tried every cosmetic cover up on the market to hide them—but nothing worked.

Trying to Recover by Staying Inside

I stayed inside more than ever before. I was trying to get better on my own. After each nursing shift I took, I was sick in bed for at least two days, sometimes even three. The fatigue was debilitating. It was interfering with my ability to earn an income. That's when I knew I was in serious trouble.

No matter how long I stayed in bed, I could not build up enough stamina for work.

Pain and Rheumatoid Arthritis

I knew that pain was a marker with lupus. It started off mild, then increased as the condition progressed. At one point, all my joints and muscles ached and often spasmed. I was diagnosed with "full blown" rheumatoid arthritis.

Sun Sensitivity

My very good dermatologist told me to avoid the sun. I hung on her every word. I stayed inside. This was no hardship, since I was so sick. It made sense to stay inside all the time.

Other Infections

I tried to ignore the fact that people with lupus are unable to fight even trivial infections. The lupus patient's immune system regulation mechanisms are weak and go haywire. So, my body would keep fighting off an infection even after the infection was long gone. Yet I was still working in the hospital ER.

Raynaud's Disease

Each time I went to see my physician, we added another diagnosis to my systemic lupus. Next, I was told I had Raynaud's disease.

Raynaud's disease makes the blood vessels in the hands and feet slam shut in the cold. It's another of the lupus body overreaction responses. When it happens, my fingers and toes turn red, white, or blue—and radiate with sharp nerve pain.

This Disease Is Relentless

As the illness progressed, I realized my case was relentless. Lupus was supposed to come and go, with periods of rest in between. So far, though, it had stayed—always active and threatening my sanity.

I was on an emotional roller-coaster that I didn't think would ever stop. The symptoms kept shifting.

I never had a chance to finish the grieving process as it dragged out with no end in sight.

Tried to Meditate

As one of my last resorts, I tried meditating, but it was too much work. I tried manufacturing positive thinking, and that felt exhausting.

Finally, I did what felt best to me. I hid. I hid because I could not figure out what was going on or how to fix it.

I knew about the stigma of seeking mental health support. I did not want to be that person.

Why would I tell everyone I need emotional support? Why share that on top of everything else?

Besides, family and friends kept saying, "You look great." *It could be better*, I wanted to say. *I am dead inside*, I should have said.

I knew that the situation I was in was my fault. I should have left my ex-husband before he walked out. I should have saved some money for therapy after the divorce. I should have prevented this disease.

I knew how this saga was going to end. My health would deteriorate, little by little. Chronic disease was going to take things from me bit by bit. Things—sports, activities—that I would never be able to do again as my symptoms worsen.

Broken Record

My mind was like a stuck record that kept repeating the same lyrics. It replayed the same dread every time I went over my past mistakes.

I continued to overthink my situation. This conjured up even more negative thoughts. The cycle continued with memories of my divorce and my parents' chronic illnesses. I felt more and more helpless—and hopeless—about the future.

This was my refrain:
Why do these things happen to me?
What's wrong with me?
Why can't I cope?
Why can't I get going?
Why do I always react this way?

～*Questions*

What illness symptoms did you have?
How did they appear?
Were you afraid?
Did you share your fears or doubts with anyone?

CHAPTER 5:
MY SECRET LIFE

When something awful happens to us, we are knee deep in regret, resentment, and mindlessness.

—Ellen Langer, PhD, Professor of Social Psychology, Harvard University

Now my days were inside the house.

When I wasn't working, I was lying in bed.

All my joints ached. They felt too worn out to find their way back to where they belonged. My bones had given up, and the muscles could care less. Together, they urged, "Stay, rest."

Getting up out of bed took preparation and time. When I did get to a standing position, I could not walk without holding onto something steady.

I couldn't read books anymore because I felt my circumstances were too serious. Things were too scary to concentrate on something other than my disease.

In my secret life, I sunk into the online lives of others with lupus. It was all I wanted to do. I joined every lupus online support group I could find. I wanted to analyze their situation and compare it with mine.

Most of the comments in these groups were anything but uplifting. People talked about medications, doctors, how awful and hopeless they felt. What kind of support was this supposed to be? I was glad that I did not know any of these people. I remained separate—apart.

"This," I said to myself, "is the beauty of online support. Nobody knows me. I don't have to explain anything to anyone. I don't have to provide support—no one will know."

So, I would lay there, scrolling through the comments. After a while, I only kept reading the comments of those who looked healthy.

Many of the members were sending each other love and prayers. I wondered if they knew each other. Or did they send love and prayers to everyone?

An Observer

I was a silent observer. I had nothing to give, nothing to offer to someone else's suffering.

After a few months, I was beginning to notice patterns. Some people were getting through the tough times and some were not.

At that time, I did not consider where I was in this mix.

Why Bother?

I had my doctor's instructions to "avoid the sun."

So, I took my medication as prescribed. If I did venture outside, I covered myself up from head to toe, no skin exposed. By the time I put on all my garb, I could not see, feel, or hear anything in the world outside my home.

So why bother? Going outside was too much trouble.

～Questions

What was your main way of surviving once you or your loved one received the scary diagnosis?

What worked, what did not?

Did you join any support groups? How did that go?

PART 2:
THE EFFECT OF
GREEN SPACE

ON WORRY, LIFESPAN, MEMORY, ATTENTION, BRAIN STRUCTURE, MOTIVATION, AND EFFORT

The land knows you, even when you are lost.
—Robin Kimmerer

Chapter 6:
One Comment

Then one day, a healthy-looking person in a lupus support group opened up my world.

She said, "When I go outside, I use tons of quality sunscreen and a hat—so far so good."

What?! That's it?! No qualifiers? No fear? So matter-of-fact.

She had systemic lupus! I wanted to be this matter of fact with my disease.

Why could she be outside? What doctor's advice was she not following? Or had she interpreted the lupus and sun sensitivity in another way? Where was her emotion?

Where was her free-floating anxiety about going outside? Where was her overwhelming fear of rampant hair loss, angry red rashes, pain, and deadly DNA damage?

What had I been doing staying inside? Had I primed myself with fear of going outside? Had I simply become a slave to imagining the worst?

I Went Outside

Full of anger at myself and my world, I decided to commit what felt like my lupus suicide.

I slapped on sunscreen, grabbed my hat, and in a rage went outside into the mid-day sun.

Under my glasses, my eyes squinted at the high noon sun. At that moment I did not care if I died out there. Life inside was no fun.

I Belonged. I Was Away.

In a flash, I felt this big black dog of depression wander off to look for something more interesting to do. I had not even noticed it there, but it had been with me all along.

Now I felt the breeze on my face. I even took my hat off in the shade. I walked. My spirits soared. My breathing slowed. I felt beautiful. I was breathing in new life.

I wanted to take long deep breaths. I drank in the air. I drew in the deep scent of the balsam fir, spruce, and jack pine.

I recognized these feelings from a time before lupus had come crashing down. No more thoughts of dread swirled around in my head. My thoughts of disease, divorce, job loss could not get a foothold on the me I found out here. I remembered the love both my parents had for the outdoors. I felt like they were walking with me.

I kept walking. The longer I walked, the better I felt. The pain in my joints eased.

As my eyes moved across the tree branches, I could feel my brain settling down.

My heart soared.

It almost felt as if the solutions to this disease were right there, in the branches of the trees.

All I had to do was get here, where I belonged.

Everything Seemed to Fit Together

My conscious mind, the one that helped me keep all my doctor's appointments straight, seemed to get out of the way. Furthermore, it moved to a place of friendly detachment toward myself.

The beauty of the natural world startled me. I noticed the way the treetops swayed in the wind. I looked deep into layers of tree branches that spread out along my path. Dead and live trees were leaning on each other. Some were creaking. The surf sounds of the treetop winds were rising and falling.

Everything seemed to fit together.

It felt like ecstasy or an endorphin flush. My body felt like a body again. Muscles found. Bones moving with new vigor.

I stayed out there in the "bush" for hours, noticing the play of light through tree branches. I ran my fingertips over spongy mosses, feeling the warmth of the sun in the pink round rock mounds. Then the feather drum of a startled partridge. I was free again and I knew it.

New Energy

On my way home, I felt as though my life was in my own hands again.

I knew what to do. My old confidence was back. I began to research what had happened to me in the woods outside.

Why was my life beautiful again after I was outside in nature?

I Could Read Again

Once I had stepped outside, I remembered my finely honed research skills. I could read again. I could concentrate on dense scientific studies.

I read hundreds of peer reviewed studies that connected nature and health.

One thing was clear to me. This was cold, hard science.

Indelible Connection Between Brain, Body, and Trees

The deeper I dug into the research, the more I realized that trees and green space have far more to do with the mind and body than anyone imagined.

Yet the indelible connection between brain, body, and trees had not reached the medical community.

In all honesty, this complex connection was just reaching me.

Uncomfortable

Although I spent my career in healthcare, I was now taking a hard left turn. This was both uncomfortable and exhilarating. It was difficult to find the research, and scary to go after it.

When I tried to talk to family, friends, and colleagues about trees they got restless and looked away. Often, they quickly agreed, "Yes, going outside is good."

But because I had not shared my specific fears of dying too fast, losing my mind, and all of my organs shutting down—we would not talk about it further. Their concern about me and the disease seemed to be all anyone could handle at the time. I understood.

I also realized that I was breaking my pattern of a nurse knowing how to work every angle of the healthcare system. They wanted to talk about that—not trees.

I had no idea where I was going with this research—except to a place of unknowing. All I knew was that going outside, close to trees, would change my mood from despair to hope in a flash.

When I did find the research, I had to write out the study methodology for myself so I could follow it and believe it. Although I had researched healthcare issues as a Professor of Nursing, I had certainly not investigated trees. I knew I was alone on this path, but I was desperate to live out my life in a different way. I followed my fears to the research on trees.

⁓Questions

At a time when you were feeling your worst, do you remember any comments that helped to move you forward?

CHAPTER 7:

CROUSE AND JAMES: LIVE LONGER WITH TREES

In general, it is best to have trees around.

We found that those who have more trees and vegetation around where they lived had an eight to 12 per cent reduced risk of (premature) dying compared to those who didn't.

—Professor Dan Crouse, health geographer, University of New Brunswick (2017)

My biggest fear at that point was dying too early. I found the recent (2017) Stanford study that headlined:

Women with systemic lupus erythematosus (SLE) in the U.S. live on average 22 years less—and men an average of 12 fewer years—than members of the same sex among the public at large, according to new data from Stanford University.

Leading causes of death for female SLE patients were septicemia (blood infections or blood poisoning) and hypertension, while male patients more often died of complications of heart disease and diabetes.

At 63 years old, I knew my time might be up. I was living on borrowed time. So I faced that fear first. I went to the tree research. It was a long shot, I knew this.

To my absolute amazement, I found evidence that would turn my "dying too early" belief around.

Professor Dan Crouse, health geographer at the University of New Brunswick, had good news for me. Along with other researchers across Canada and the United States, Crouse studied 1.3 million Canadians in 30 cities over an 11-year period.

The study used data from the 2001 long-form census and compared it to the Canadian mortality database for the next 11 years. They measured the amount of greenery from trees, shrubs, grass, and other plants within 250 metres (about two blocks) of the study subjects' homes, using postal codes and satellite data.

They found that having daily exposure to trees and other greenery can extend a person's life. His study found that as the amount of greenery increased, people's risk of premature death from natural causes decreased "significantly." "There was a lot bigger effect than I think any of us had been expecting."

Nurses with and Without Chronic Disease

The research team led by Dr. Dan Crouse at the University of New Brunswick had good news. They found that living within two blocks of green space makes you live longer.

More and more research proved the correlation between life spans and surrounding tree areas. University research teams spent decades following where and how long people lived. The results? Trees always made the difference in people's longevity. I could hardly believe my eyes.

And then I found a study that included women (nurses) with chronic diseases.

Trees Help Us Live Longer with Chronic Disease

A nationwide Harvard University study investigated the role trees play on patients with and without chronic disease. In 2017, the results were published.

In this study, Harvard researchers followed where nurses lived over a 43-year time period.

Professor Peter James and his team of Epidemiology and Environmental Health scientists at Harvard discovered that those women whose home was surrounded by trees and green spaces lived longer.

The 100,000+ women (with and without chronic disease) who had greenness within a 15-minute walk radius of their homes had a 12% lower early death rate than those who lived in the least green areas.

How They Did It

This study started in 1976 with 121,701 women who were registered nurses ages 30–55 and were from 11 states.

For 43 years (so far), researchers at Harvard have followed this same process:

"Twice a year nurses state their medical diagnosis and their health exposures."

The study defined health exposures as: air pollution, noise, and extreme heat.

The nurses' response rates for their surveys were 90%. The researchers calculated the response rate in the study as the number of women who returned the survey and were still alive.

A major strength of this study was the use of sophisticated satellite imagery from NASA's Terra satellite. This allowed the team to measure the detail of greenness around each study participant's residence, which included a radius reachable in a 10–15-minute walk outside the home.

I Would Be Around to See New Trees Grow

Going through this research I was winning back years of my life. I felt so hopeful that I planted a vegetable garden for the first time in 20 years. And I planted trees—eight of them—in my back yard. I knew that I would be around to see them grow. I tried not to talk about trees too much with friends and family. I felt better that way. But I did spend most of my time planting and watering trees.

Through this lifespan research I came back to life and even remembered my healthy habit of going to the gym.

My Fitness Classes

I knew the classes in Pine Falls would offer more than fitness. Indeed, they became my social fix. My next-door neighbour and I would walk along the tree-lined street to my old high school gym at 6:20 a.m. three times a week.

There we would meet a group of 15 women whom we've known forever, all going through something. We would smile and joke our way through gruelling exercises.

This was how I got stronger for going outside. And I was there because I had stepped outside. I found new courage. New hope.

∽Questions

Have you thought about going outside as a way to live longer?

Do you live within a 15-minute walk to green space (grass, trees, gardens, backyard, or park)?

In what ways can you plan daily exposure to green space?

Would you try to make a list of your friends who like to be outside?

What opportunities do you have to go to fitness classes or the gym to stay fit for the outdoors?

CHAPTER 8:
BRATMAN AND NOLEN-HOEKSEMA: OUTSIDE AND OVERTHINKING

Negative rumination is repetitive thought focused on negative aspects of the self. The behavior shows up as increased activity in the subgenual prefrontal cortex, a narrow band that regulates negative emotions.

> —Greg Bratman, when he was a doctoral student in the Emmett Interdisciplinary Program in Environment and Resources and the Center for Conservation Biology, Stanford University

Negative rumination is repeatedly thinking about the causes or consequences of problems without moving to active problem-solving.

Negative rumination not only interferes with people's ability to solve problems but their ability to obtain help from others.

> —Susan Nolen-Hoeksema, PhD, psychologist, Yale University

Overthinking

Before my research into the matter of trees and chronic disease, I had thought I was the only person who constantly replayed in her mind the upsetting situations from the past. My thoughts easily obsessed around my divorce, my disease, and my parents' chronic illnesses.

Then, to my surprise—and joy—I learned that there is a name for this type of thinking: rumination. It is emotional regulation gone haywire.

Basically, I was a ruminator.

When I was ruminating, I often had thoughts like these go through my mind:

"Why do these things happen to me?"

"What's wrong with me?"

"I should be able to cope with this."

"Why can't I stop overeating?"

Ruminating Can Lead to Binge-Eating

Easy to understand research on rumination was conducted by Yale University psychologist Susan Nolen-Hoeksema, PhD. (Sadly, Nolen-Hoeksema died in 2013 at the age of 53, following heart surgery and a blood infection.)

According to Susan Nolen-Hoeksema, rumination is associated with a variety of negative consequences, including anxiety, depression, substance use, and binge-eating. She is the author of the book *Eating, Drinking, Overthinking*, where she explains how these issues develop.

Nolen-Hoeksema is also the author of *Women Who Think Too Much: How to Break Free of Overthinking and Reclaim Your Life*. She lets us off the hook a little when she says ruminators may simply have more stress in their lives which preoccupies them.

She also states: "Some people prone to ruminate have basic problems pushing things out of consciousness once they get there." So, according to her words, women tend to be more concerned about their relationships. Since ambiguities abound in those environments, Hoeksema says "interpersonal relationships are great fuel for rumination."

According to Nolen-Hoeksema, "you can never really know what people think of you or whether they will be faithful and true."

Her research fits with my case. I had no idea that I was a ruminator. I did not go for help to family or friends. While I was hiding inside, I was ruminating on my chronic illness, my divorce, and the loss of my parents to their chronic conditions.

Since I had no idea that I had become a ruminator during my marriage, I did not discuss this with anyone. I certainly didn't know whether a solution existed. It was not until I stepped into the trees, taking my chronic disease along, that I found the solution I had been yearning for.

If only I had known that Stanford University scientists had already had the answer back in 2015. I could have been free much sooner. It could have been remarkably easy.

Landmark Stanford University Study: Going Outside Takes Rumination Away

In 2015, Stanford's Gregory Bratman and his team conducted a groundbreaking study which showed that when ordinary people (with no history of mental illness) went outside, two things happened:
— One, rumination decreased and went away.
— Two, activity in the subgenual prefrontal cortex of the brain decreased.

The subgenual prefrontal cortex is the part of the brain that registers negative thoughts or rumination. It's a breakthrough that those scientists managed to find a way to measure the effects of trees/green space on our thoughts and emotions.

How They Did It

For this study, published in *Proceedings of the National Academy of Sciences*, the Stanford team examined whether a nature walk could reduce rumination in 38 people with no history of mental disorder.

They intentionally picked city dwellers and had them walk in the area around Stanford University, near San Francisco. Half the participants walked for 90 minutes in grassland with oak trees and shrubs and distant views of San Francisco Bay. The other half took a stroll along a four-lane highway, right by the El Camino Real, in Palo Alto.

Brain Scans

Brain scans were performed both before and after the walk. This allowed the researchers to track the activity in the participants' subgenual prefrontal cortex—which the study calls, "an area that has been shown to be particularly active during the type of maladaptive, self-reflective thought and behavioral withdrawal that occurs during rumination."

Before and after the walk, the participants were asked to complete a survey that was used to measure their inward thinking.

Among the survey items were: "My attention is often focused on aspects of myself I wish I'd stop thinking about," and, "I spend a great deal of time thinking back over my embarrassing or disappointing moments."

The results showed that those participants who had walked in urban green space for 90 minutes answered the survey differently after their walk. Their rumination—and their brain activity in the subgenual prefrontal cortex—had decreased.

The urban walkers, on the other hand, showed no improvements either in the survey or the brain scan.

I Am a Ruminator

I could not believe my eyes. I had just discovered that I was a ruminator—and now I actually had the solution in my hands. It was easy. It was freeing. I could do this.

The research showed me that going outside to be close to trees is a simple strategy to feel empowered. For me, this information became the difference between living life to the fullest and waiting around to die.

Negative Rumination Questions

If you would like to examine your own thought process, here are some questions (direct quotes) from Dr. Susan Nolen-Hoeksema's Rumination Survey:

— Do you often reflect on episodes of your life that you should no longer concern yourself with?
— Do you often focus on aspects of yourself you wish you would stop thinking about?
— Do you always seem to be rehashing things you've said or done?
— Is it sometimes hard to turn off thoughts about yourself?
— Long after a disagreement or argument is concluded, do your thoughts keep going back to what happened?
— Are you often playing back in your mind how you acted in a past situation?
— Is it easy for you to put unwanted thoughts out of your mind?
— Do you spend a great deal of time thinking back over embarrassing or disappointing moments?
— Do you find your thoughts are focused on things that are not going well, instead of seeing the larger picture?
— Are your recurring thoughts related to your personal relationships?
— When are you most likely to overthink?
— Do you binge eat, binge drink, or have addictions? Could these be related to overthinking?

CHAPTER 9:
BRATMAN AND NOLEN-HOEKSEMA: ADAPTIVE SELF-REFLECTION

This field is new, and there's a lot of work to be done. But we can say, with some degree of certainty, that in many cases nature experience benefits mood and cognitive function (and likely emotion regulation as well, although that is less studied).

> —Greg Bratman, (former Stanford University Negative Rumination Study lead author) Professor of Nature, Health and Recreation in the School of Environmental and Forest Sciences at the University of Washington. He also works at EarthLab's Nature for Health—a group of collaborators that work to put science into practice in ways that benefit underserved and other populations.

I learned that rumination, although it has us contemplating past mistakes, is not the same as self-examination. Indeed, overthinking offers no new insights while it intensifies our negative feelings.

This unhealthy inward thinking makes us become narrowly focused on the things that are not going well instead of seeing the larger picture.

So much of my head space had been filled with rumination, I wondered how, moving forward, I could teach myself to think in a healthy way.

It wasn't difficult to notice that being outside created some distance from my negative thoughts. I was able to roll them over, examine them, reflect on them, and explore new ideas. I knew this was the healthy way to do it.

I Learned About Adaptive Self-Reflection

Nolen-Hoeksema had also studied a concept opposite of rumination: adaptive self-reflection. When people practice adaptive self-reflection, they focus on the concrete parts of a situation and the improvements they can make. For instance, a person may wonder, "What exactly am I worried about?"

After pouring over Bratman's rumination study and Susan Nolen-Hoeksema's work, I learned that reflecting on issues is a good, productive activity. It is only when I keep thinking the same thought over and over again that the process becomes unhelpful.

Lesson Learned: Able to Be Kind to Myself and Others

When I went outside near trees, I was able to recognize my fears. My anger had piled on top of my fears. I saw my own excruciating vulnerability and loss of control. I saw how easy it had been to nurture my chronic disease loss list.

Now I recognized this as faulty thinking and brain activity in my subgenual prefrontal cortex. Going outside gave me new control. I was in the driver's seat of my thoughts. I allowed my brain to "recalculate" my whereabouts, just as on my car GPS. I did not judge my thoughts. I saw them with detached interest.

I began to care about myself. I told myself, "It is going to be OK." I pretended I was talking to my boys. I stopped fighting. I stopped complicating my thinking. I was able to be kind to those around me and in my life. It was easy. This felt right.

I started commenting in my lupus support groups. I thanked the group member who inspired me to go outside.

I was back in love with my world. Only this time I felt so free.

When the old negative thoughts surfaced, I said to myself, "There's that neurological glitch again; I can ignore that." I had a new tool.

Stepping outside was like a whole new bandwidth that opened up in my mind. By stepping outside I opened up my heart to myself and to others. I no longer felt so hurt. I could shift my thinking. I could push unwanted thoughts out of my mind. I was free.

Goodbye Binge Eating

The research on repetitive negative thought cycles and the effects of green space on mood showed me the connection with my binge eating. It was the rumination. Prior to this evidence, I felt shame that I could not control my impulsive eating. Now I was aware that the eating was tied to the neurological glitch of overthinking. Now I understood the root cause of this behavior.

I forgave myself. I was able to see binge eating for what it was: my response to negative rumination. I had new insight. I could find my way out of this pattern. It was as easy as stepping outside. Goodbye, negative thought cycles, and goodbye, binge eating! Hello, tree branches. I began to see the mind-body-tree connection. I began to live it.

∼Questions

Is it easier for you to get unwanted thoughts out of your mind when you are outside?

Is it easier for you to reflect on your circumstances when you are outside?

When you are worried about something, can you ask yourself, "What exactly am I worried about?"

When you are not overthinking, do you find it easier to be gentler with yourself and others?

CHAPTER 10:
BERMAN AND BRATMAN: MAY I HAVE YOUR ATTENTION PLEASE?

Natural environments filled with intriguing stimuli, modestly grab the attention in a bottom-up fashion, allowing top-down directed-attention abilities a chance to replenish.

Unlike natural environments, urban environments are filled with stimulation that captures the attention dramatically and additionally requires directed attention (e.g., to avoid being hit by a car), making them less restorative.

—Professor Marc Berman, an Industrial Engineer and Professor in the Department of Psychology, University of Chicago. His research interests lie in the "ability of natural environments to improve affect, attention, and memory." He received post-doctoral training at the University of Toronto's Rotman Research Institute at Baycrest.

May I Have Your Attention, Please?

Thanks to Stanford scientist Gregory Bratman, I now know that a brief walk in urban green spaces puts a break on a person's negative thought patterns. Spending time in grassy areas with trees around you changes your mindset.

But that's not all Bratman did. Next, his team showed that walking in urban green space "improved cognition." Cognition, in their study, referred to our short- and long-term memory, our ability to concentrate, problem-solve, and learn new things.

Refresh Your Brain

After conducting his study, Bratman, now a professor at the School of Environmental and Forest Sciences, University of Washington, concluded that interactions with nature not only reduce human stress, but also "enhance the restoration of directed attention." In other words, being in nature helps us to be more tuned in to the present moment; it allows us to pay attention to life.

Says Bratman in 2018, "This field is new, and there's a lot of work to be done. But we can say, with some degree of certainty, that in many cases nature experience benefits mood and cognitive function (and likely emotion regulation as well, although that is less studied)."

Bratman's work ties in with other researchers. Professor Marc Berman at the University of Chicago did his post-doctoral work in the Toronto area.

Improve Your Concentration

Marc Berman is an Engineer with a PhD in Psychology and a Professor at the University of Chicago. Berman further explored the subject of attention abilities and concentration. In his studies he found that walking in—or simply looking at images of—green spaces refreshes our brain and improves our attention.

Berman's research showed that a 50-minute walk in nature improves short-term memory by 20%, while no significant gains were reported after an urban walk.

His research team found similar memory improvement results when participants simply viewed pictures of nature vs. urban scenes. Both viewings were conducted in quiet experiment rooms.

Mental Energy Is Needed to "Pay Attention"

Researchers who perform these studies say that our brains need mental energy in order to "pay attention." They also state that mental energy is limited—and goes up and down. When our mental energy level is too low, we experience mental fatigue.

In his study, Berman found that green spaces restore mental energy and our attention. According to his results, trees and urban green space give us energy to pay attention.

So, when we are tired of paying attention (mental fatigue), trees and green space boost our mental energy. When our mental energy levels are high, we can pay attention. Scientists call this observation the Attention Restoration Theory (ART).

Science is becoming more and more interested in the role nature plays in restoring our attention once we have experienced mental fatigue.

Lupus Brain Fog

A symptom of lupus is "brain fog." This is defined as the inability to pay attention, and it's a symptom that greatly interferes with my ability to perform mental tasks. For example, writing is difficult when I cannot pay attention to my own work. It often feels like my brain has gone off to a nap somewhere.

For this reason, I had my own questions about paying attention. I wondered: "Can I get my attention to come back when I need it?" And, "How does green space work on my attention?" I had new hope about the possibility to clear my brain fog. I was over the moon with the following study results.

Natural Environments Grab Your Attention

When you are outside you pay attention in a different way. Brain and cognition researchers at the University of Amsterdam explain the different ways of paying attention this way:

Bottom-up attention is when you notice anything once you step outside. Your attention automatically goes there. This attention is automatic and involuntary and happens instantly.

Top-down attention takes more time and concentration. It's under your clear control. This is the attention required to write a sentence or drive your car.

Your Mind Can Wander in Green Space

In green space where trees grow, you don't have to pay direct attention to your surroundings. When in nature, your mind can wander about and softly focus on each detail. This kind of attention is not all-consuming.

So, when you go outside and your mind wanders around, you are giving your brain a gift. You are giving your brain a break.

I now schedule five-minute outside breaks every 90 minutes. I step outside and take 3 deep breaths. It really works.

Green Space Restores Your Ability to Pay Attention…

Berman's study showed that walking outside in urban green space as well as looking at pictures of nature gives us back the energy required to pay attention in our everyday lives.

Scientists call this the "restorative value" of green space on attention.

… And You Become More Cheerful

At the University of Glasgow, the Department of Psychology conducted a similar study called "An investigation into the restorative effects of the outdoors on undergraduate students."

The university was looking at ways to help students cope with the common problem of long hours of studying.

Consequently, their aim was to investigate the effects of green space on well-being, attention, and other cognitive abilities in undergraduate students.

According to the results, the participants who experienced the outdoors intervention (as opposed to the indoor intervention) were happier afterwards. They were also able to pay attention to their studies for a longer time.

In the study, well-being and happiness items included statements on optimism, usefulness, relaxation, interest, confidence, cheerfulness, and energy.

Of all the items, "cheerfulness" had the highest increase post-test.

How They Did It

When conducting the indoor and outdoor study, the researchers asked a sample of 30 participants to complete three tasks:

1) fill in a well-being questionnaire pre- and post-environmental intervention;
2) perform a computer task;
3) carry out a learning task.

These were directly followed by an indoor or outdoor environment visit. The indoor setting was quiet and calm.

Below are some of the statements included in the well-being questionnaire. The participants had to indicate to what extent they agreed with each statement before and after the test:

— I am feeling optimistic about the future.
— I am feeling relaxed.
— I am feeling interested in other people.
— I am thinking clearly.
— I am feeling good about myself.
— I am feeling closer to other people.
— I am feeling confident.
— I am able to make up my own mind about things.
— I am feeling loved.
— I am feeling cheerful.

I Began to Write

After spending more and more time outside, I was able to focus on writing. This was something I had hoped to do for years but could not find the discipline for it. It turned out that discipline was not the issue—concentration was. Every time I came in from having spent time outside, my mind was clear and ready to focus on writing.

∼Questions

When does your ability to pay attention go up or down?

How much of your day requires concentration (top-down attention) e.g., driving, writing, working?

Can you schedule an outside micro break around your deep concentration times?

Have you noticed whether you can pay attention more easily once you have been outside?

Do you find that your attention can wander when you are outside?

Chapter 11:
Berman: Healthy Tree, Healthy Me

Having 11 more average-sized trees per city block resulted in decreased disease conditions. This equates to a $20,200 increase in income along with gaining 1.4 years to one's life.

—Marc Berman

As I continued digging for more information on urban green space research, I wanted to run outside and yell from my roof top: "We're going to be ok! We've got this! Hallelujah."

I liked Berman's work and stayed with his projects.

The next study of his I found sounded too good to be true. It stated that spending time around trees decreases disease, makes us live longer, reduces stress, and makes us feel richer.

And you don't have to move to the forest to get the benefits. All these studies were done in urban green spaces—city parks with grass and trees.

Toronto Trees

Building on his previous research which showed that interaction with urban green space is good for the brain, psychologist Marc Berman at the University of Chicago turned his attention to city trees.

Berman, who did his post-doctoral work in Toronto, returned to the city because it offers several important data sets for the same areas, including:

— detailed maps and satellite photos of the "urban forest;"
— maps showing household income by area;
— and the continuing Ontario Health Study, a survey conducted on 31,000 people from more than 3,000 neighborhoods—which they could overlay on the tree maps.

The survey included questions on heart disease, stroke, diabetes, obesity, cancer, depression, and addiction. It also asked people to assess their own overall state of health.

How They Did It

The research team studied 530,000 trees along the streets in Toronto and analyzed them by location, species, and diameter. These were trees people saw around the places they live, work, and shop and could easily view through a window.

The team then combined their findings with satellite images of trees growing in people's backyards. Finally, the researchers compared the number of trees to the health of people on each block, controlling for income, age, and education so the results were not influenced by these variables.

Trees Make You Healthy, Wealthy, and Happy

By studying the tree canopies in Toronto, in combination with 30,000 health surveys, the researchers found that people who live in neighborhoods with a higher density of trees report decreased disease, increased life expectancy, and higher net worth.

Specifically, having 11 more average-sized trees per city block resulted in decreased disease conditions. The researchers said that this equates to "a $20,200 increase in income" along with gaining 1.4 years to one's life.

Additionally, the research team found that the health of people in poorer neighborhoods with lots of trees matched the health of those in wealthier treed neighborhoods. The reverse was also true: the health of richer people who lived in areas without large trees matched the health of people in poorer city communities that lacked vegetation.

I Did Feel Richer

When I sold my mortgage-free Burlington, Ontario, home and moved to my hometown of Pine Falls, Manitoba, I did feel richer. I also felt happier and healthier than I had in decades.

This little town is in the boreal forest along the Winnipeg River. I could not have found a better place to live. I was home.

My children and loved ones, however, still lived in cities, but I was hopeful because this research was conducted in Toronto. So, as long as they could get out to green spaces, they would be ok.

But I needed to open their eyes to this research. I decided to start a blog and website to get the word about trees out. I called it TreesMendUs.com.

~Questions

Are there trees (even one) within walking distance of where you live?

If not, are there other ways you can get to urban green space?

Do you feel healthier, happier, and richer when you are in green space with trees?

Chapter 12:
Ulrich: What You See
Is What You Get

What if you can't get outside? Simply looking at an image of nature works, too. You can either observe nature from a window, or view a picture of it, both of which elicit fast responses in our brain and have positive effects on our mind and body.

The technical jargon for this phenomenon is the "importance of visual access to green space." Looking at a picture of nature or at the tree outside your window are both examples of "micro-restorative activities."

I remembered my dad with MS sitting in his wheelchair. When he could not be outside, and especially in the winter, he loved his station at our huge tree-filled living room windows. He simply enjoyed his "visual access to green space." We didn't have that name for it then, but the results were the same. My dad was recovering from the stress of life with MS by looking outside into trees.

Stress Recovery Faster with Image of Nature

Ahead of his time, in the 70's and 80's, Roger Ulrich, a young psychologist in Michigan, did brain EEGs (electroencephalograms) on study participants while they first looked at pictures of nature and then at pictures of buildings.

In the first instance, the participants showed higher alpha wave activity, associated with relaxation and increased serotonin production.

After the brain measures, Ulrich performed cardiovascular measures: heart rate and pulse rate transit time (time it takes to change heart rate).

For one of his studies, Ulrich's 120 subjects first viewed a stressful movie and then watched videos of nature or urban settings. Basically, Ulrich wanted to learn more about stress recovery and what showed up in the body after a stressful event.

Through his research, Ulrich found that stress recovery and transition to a positive mood happened faster and more completely when the subjects viewed natural scenery. These alterations in mood were matched by positive changes in the subjects' physiological activity levels (heart rate) and an increased ability to concentrate. In fact, the heart rate slowed minutes after exposure to a natural environment.

Looking at Images of Nature Provides a Buffer for Future Stress

Interestingly, Ulrich also found that viewing natural scenery provided a buffer for future stress. He called this the effect of nature "on stress recovery and stress immunization." Basically, looking at images of trees not only relieves stress at the time, but it eases future stress as well.

The Tree Outside Your Window

Then, in 1984, came his famous study on the view through a hospital window. According to Ulrich's findings, surgical patients assigned to rooms with a window looking out on trees spent less days in the hospital after surgery, healed quicker, had less pain, and took fewer analgesics than the patients in rooms with windows facing a brick wall.

You Want Lots of Parasympathetic Activity

The body's response to trees and green space is largely run by the autonomic nervous system (ANS) which is divided into the sympathetic and the parasympathetic branches. The sympathetic side regulates the fight-flight response by increasing the heart rate, heart pumping (myocardial contractility), and sweating.

The parasympathetic branch, on the other hand, causes slowing of the heart, more variable heart rate, and increased saliva production. This is the system that kicks in to help us recover from stress and buffer us from future anxiety. We want lots of parasympathetic activity. Here's why.

In 2013, professors Daniel Brown and Jo Barton of the School of Biological Sciences at the University of Essex published "Viewing Nature Scenes Positively Affects Recovery of Autonomic Function Following Acute-Mental Stress."

In this landmark study, Brown and Barton found that para-sympathetic activity (the resting one) was higher after looking at nature compared to looking at scenes of built environments. According to their findings, within just the first five minutes of viewing nature scenes, the participants showed signs of parasympathetic recovery.

Naturally, this benchmark study laid the groundwork for similar research.

In 2015, Magdalena van den Berg at the University Medical Centre in Amsterdam looked at stress recovery and published: "Autonomic Nervous System Responses to Viewing Green and Built Settings: Differentiating Between Sympathetic and Parasympathetic Activity."

How They Did It

This study involved 46 students who were shown photos of green or built spaces before, and immediately after, a stressful situation—in this case, an important exam. The students' heart rates and heart pumping patterns were recorded at these same times by EKG (electrocardiogram).

The study showed that five minutes of viewing urban green space supported recovery from stress. The students that looked at photos of green spaces after the exam had lower heart rates five minutes later. It took much longer for the students that looked at pictures of built spaces to get back to a normal heart rate.

Green Spaces: A Buffer Against Future Stress

Like Ulrich, van den Berg's studies also showed that exposure to real or simulated green space not only promotes recovery from stress, but also acts as a buffer against the negative impact of future stressful life events.

Bank Stress Resilience

By the time I found this research, I knew all about stress, and it is no surprise that I wanted to protect myself from similar future experiences. Could I bank stress resilience?

The physician who has been coordinating my care is a rheumatologist, which means constant referrals to other specialists and numerous tests that often show some new deterioration. To keep my mind above the abyss that those test results could pull me into, I had to find a buffer. That's what I recognized the outside does for me. When I am in nature, I feel magnificent. When I am inside, I am fine—except when I am not, and then I sleep.

When I start to ruminate over my test results, I step outside. It works. I draw in deep breaths of tree aerosols and relief.

Rheumatoid Arthritis and Walking Poles

I have both lupus and rheumatoid arthritis. When I first started walking in the woods, I wanted a stick to scare away stray dogs. No dogs so far, but I can't begin to count how many times my walking poles have saved me from going down. And now I find they are irreplaceable.

I trip uphill, downhill, on flats, on rough, and on the smooth. Each time I trip I catch myself with my poles; I also use them to prod suspect footing before I take a step. On the uneven forest floor, hiking poles keep me balanced. They keep me upright and give me a good walking posture. They take the pressure off my sore hips and knees. The poles became my rehab support. I started to search for poles designed by physiotherapists. I found some and ordered them online.

The Canadian company Urban Poling, developed by a physiotherapist and an occupational therapist, operates like a non-profit. Their poles are used by people with Arthritis, Parkinson's, and MS and are specially designed with added edge on the handles to provide more support and lift than others I have tried.

I wish that my father who'd suffered from MS could have used these poles. I remember trying hard, together as a family, to push past the embarrassment and shame we shared as he bravely used one cane for the first time. He was in his 40's. Soon, the one cane was followed by another. He could have had a period of no humiliation. He could have been walking with Nordic walking poles. He could have been seen as a European cross-country skier in off-season training. We could have joined him with no stigma. It could have been so much better for him.

~Questions

Have you noticed what happens to you if you look at an image of nature for 5 minutes after a stressful event?

What happens to you when you look out the window into green space for 5 minutes? (Research calls this a "micro restorative activity" that reduces stress). Think about how you might use this simple activity as a tool for your "stress immunization" or a way of buffering yourself from future stress.

Have you heard of the benefits of Nordic walking (lifting pressure off your knees and hips, providing balance)?

Do you know that walking poles may be considered rehabilitation devices—used instead of canes or walkers?

Do you know that if a doctor writes you a prescription for rehabilitation, these may be covered under your health insurance plan?

CHAPTER 13:
SCOTT AND KUHN: YOUR BRAIN AND STRESS

Managing stress is not just about feeling better in the moment, it is about protecting ourselves from losing our mental capacity.

An interdisciplinary team of researchers in the fields of aging, behavioral sciences, neurological sciences, and nursing collaborated on a study that built on existing research on aging, stress, and brain function.

Stress Affects the Way Older Adults Pay Attention and Problem-Solve

As I searched, I discovered that long-term stress affects how our brains work. Studies show that chronic stress may contribute to "cognitive loss and dementia." This was enough to capture my attention. My mother was a worrier. She did everything else right. She was fit and healthy. Could her patterns of rumination have led to her mental demise in her 60's and 70's?

The stress and aging studies, particularly those involving chronic disease, show that both affect our "cognitive function"— the way we remember, learn, problem-solve, and pay attention.

Stacey Scott, professor in Aging Studies at the University of South Florida, and Jennifer Graham-Engeland, professor in Behavioral Health at Penn State, led the study. It was funded by the National Centre of Advancing Translational Science and aimed to assess the impact of stress on older adults' "age-related cognitive loss."

This team showed that unconstructive repetitive thought (URT), or negative rumination, can take away your attention. And if this URT pattern happens for too long it can affect the body and lead to inflammation. This state, in turn, may lead to loss of memory, problem-solving ability, and concentration.

In this national study stress is defined as fear and anxiety based in "early adversity, chronic strains, major events, and daily hassles." The team cite the large body of research that shows stress can affect our cognitive function in the short- and long-term.

This same study profiles research that shows stress increases when your thoughts are occupied by past arguments or repetitive thoughts of disappointing or embarrassing moments. These are called "unconstructive thought patterns," or negative rumination, and were addressed by the landmark Stanford study that showed rumination goes away once we step outside into urban green space.

The negative thought cycles of rumination "result in our reduced ability to pay attention, keep track of, or remember steps in the task at hand." So, stress leads to rumination, and rumination leads to impairment of our ability to learn, pay attention, and problem-solve.

Stress May Increase the Risk of Dementia

This multi-field research team state that stress over the long term results in "cognitive decline compared to less-stressed peers at the same age."

Cognitive decline is a term referring to short- and long-term memory loss and dementia.

According to research profiled in this study, when you are thinking about stressful past events and situations, you are overusing your cognitive resources or brain power. This, in turn, drains the amount of brain power left for non-stressful times.

This research also shows that stress causes more inflammation and negative mood, both of which are connected to fatigue and hence affect the amount and quality of the attention we can pay to other things.

In the course of our life span, chronic life stress, as the research shows, affects our ability to learn, remember, and pay attention. Moreover, stress speeds up this loss of cognitive function while increasing our chances of dementia.

Over the long term, chronic life stress has been consistently associated with poorer cognitive function, accelerated cognitive decline, and increased incidence of dementia.

Managing stress is not just about feeling better in the moment, it is about protecting ourselves from losing our mental capacity.

This is how Scott describes their project:

> *A key objective of the ESCAPE (Effects of Stress on Cognitive Aging, Physiology, and Emotion) project is to evaluate whether engaging in stress-related unconstructive repetitive thought (URT) is a pathway through which stressful experiences negatively affect cognitive health over the short- and long-term.*
>
> *Over the short-term, we hypothesize that engaging in URT will deplete attentional resources and result in worse cognitive performance in daily life. Over the long-term, we expect that the effects of chronic stress, from repeated exposure to stressors and regular engagement in URT, will be apparent in dysregulated hypothalamic-pituitary-adrenal (HPA) axis function and inflammation. Over time, stress-related physiological dysregulation will result in accelerated cognitive decline.*

As the 2015 study Bratman conducted at Stanford shows, being outside in urban green space takes away those "unconstructive thought patterns." You could see this in your brain scan. The activity in your subgenual prefrontal cortex would decrease. By stepping outside you will have performed your own medical procedure. As a result, you will be better equipped to control your thoughts, your mindset, and your chronic disease process.

Your Brain Can Grow and Change at Any Age

Research on brain plasticity supports the assumption that the environment can shape brain structure and function. That is why we are interested in the environmental conditions that may have positive effects on brain development.

—Professor of Neuroplasticity, Simone Kuhn, Max Planck Institute

As I was digging further into all published sources, curious to discover the mystery of my positive mindset near trees, I found more and more evidence about the impact of tree proximity on the biology of the brain and the state of our mind. The connection was far stronger than anyone imagined.

Recent research by Martin Lövdén, Aging Research Center, Karolinska Institute & Stockholm University, Sweden, and Center for Lifespan Psychology, Max Planck Institute for Human Development, Berlin, Germany, shows that our brain has the ability to grow and change throughout life—even as we age. So, although you may be in your 60's, 70's, 80's, or even 90's, your brain can grow.

Simone Kuhn, Professor of Neuroplasticity at the Max Planck Institute in Germany, uses images of the brain to show that "the brain has the capacity to increase the breath of its function with age."

Kuhn's work explains further that, indeed, "various insults of aging occur" (shrinkage, white matter lesions) but the brain responds by "expanding function and perhaps growing additional tissue in response to extensive usage. This is the essence of neuroplasticity—the brain's ability to respond and adapt to its changing circumstances."

This alteration caused by life experience is called brain neuroplasticity. Neuroplasticity is defined as the way our brain forms new cells and neural connections and improves its capabilities throughout life.

According to new research sources, the environment can shape brain structure and function—all through our lives.

Age does not matter when it comes to your brain plasticity.

Older City Dwellers MRI Study Shows Healthier Stress-Processing Brain Regions

In 2017, a study was conducted by the Max Planck Institute in Germany looking at the brains of older Berliners, ages 61 to 82 years, to learn more about the connection between brain biology and tree proximity.

The research team, led by psychologist Simone Kühn, studied the environments near people's homes, focusing on the effects of forest, urban green, or wasteland on the stress-processing brain regions.

The main stress-reducing part of the brain is the almond-sized amygdala. This part of the brain plays a key role in processing your emotions, including fear and anxiety.

According to their study, those city dwellers living closer to a forest or wooded area were more likely to show a "physiologically healthy amygdala structure." To keep their objectivity, they also supposed that people with biologically bigger amygdala may have moved to treed areas—but the team didn't think that was the case, given the odds.

The researchers hence concluded that because the amygdala was bigger in these older adults, "they were therefore presumably better able to cope with stress." This effect remained stable when differences in educational qualifications and income levels were controlled for.

The study further showed that urban dwellers who lived within a one-kilometer radius of a forest had structural brain changes that positively affected their mental capabilities.

The forest, the researchers concluded, "enhances the activation of certain brain areas." The main affected brain area was the amygdala—the central nucleus in the brain that plays a key role in processing emotions, including fear and anxiety.

How They Did It

The 341 participants in Kühn's study fell between the ages of 61 and 82 years. During the study, the team was particularly interested in the "structure of the stress-processing brain regions, especially the amygdala." They used magnetic resonance imaging (MRI) to assess and examine the influence of nature's proximity to peoples' homes on this brain region.

The researchers then combined the MRI data with geoinformation about the participants' places of residence and found a "positive association between the coverage of forest and amygdala integrity."

According to the study results, those city dwellers living close to a forest showed a healthy amygdala structure. This, Kühn's team suggested, helps these city dwellers to better cope with stress, defined as: "early adversity, chronic strains, major events, and daily hassles."

My Mother Had Dementia

My mother was kind, beautiful, and competent. She also worried too much that she had said or done the wrong thing a day, a week, or a month in the past. These were always little things, but they concerned her.

Then she happily looked after my father when he was grounded by multiple sclerosis. The trauma of losing your beloved husband day by day to a degenerative disease must have been a chronic stressor. We did not know then that stress was among the major causes of cognitive decline.

∽Questions

Try to make the connection between your time spent in green space and your cognitive function. Notice before and after going outside, your differences in:
— short-term and long-term memory
— learning abilities
— problem-solving abilities
— concentration.

Make the connection between "unconstructive repeating thoughts" in your life and these cognitive abilities.

Do you live within a one-kilometer walk to trees or greenery?

Have you noticed that your brain might be finding it easier to deal with fear, anxiety, and worry if you live near green space?

What happens to your thoughts when you step outside?

CHAPTER 14:
BERESFORD-KROEGER:
YOUR FOREST PHARMACY

Trees are chemical factories that can save our lives.

...trees release unseen medicinal compounds in the form of aerosols, like rockets into the air.

...natural chemical substances float down from the tree crowns.

All wood of trees releases medically active aerosols in minute amounts. Once these chemicals are airborne, they can travel great distances. Here they may release themselves as potent antibiotic, antibacterial, anti-fungal, or anti-inflammatory shield in the air from the tropics to the poles.

The atmosphere around trees may be the most powerful natural medicine we have access to, yet most of us are completely unaware of it.

> —Diana Beresford-Kroeger, a Canadian botanist, lecturer, and medical researcher in the fields of botany, medical biochemistry, organic chemistry, and nuclear chemistry

Diana Beresford-Kroeger gives us new reasons to get close enough to pick up the scent of a tree.

At this point in my search, I needed a break from scientific papers. I needed a wider view of the forest. I wanted someone who could use science to give me new insight into trees.

Now in her 70's, Diana Beresford-Kroeger thinks broadly about science and medicine. She is a visionary scientist.

Beresford-Kroeger was among the first, along with Dr. Li in Japan, to talk about the bioactive substances, or aerosols, that trees release into the air.

When we are close to trees, we can breathe in the health giving aerosols their leaves, pine needles, bark, shrubs, bushes, mosses, ferns, and even soil emit.

Beresford-Kroeger explains that trees contain terpene oils, a natural repellent for mammals and insects that might feed on them. Since they cannot run away from danger, trees give off tiny molecules to protect themselves. To us, these chemicals are like natural medicines that we can benefit from just by breathing when surrounded by trees.

When I learned this, my view of the woods changed. Now when I enter the woods, I feel like I am joining up with a large, living and breathing circle of ancestors. I become part of it.

Trees Hold the Answers to Health and Medicine

Beresford-Kroeger grows rare trees in her garden. She has compiled the master plans to create a living library of tree DNA. In her lectures, she stresses the importance of planting one tree a year for six years.

Trees, she says, have more complex genetic structure than humans do. Moreover, people and trees have co-existed for millions of years.

According to Beresford-Kroeger, forests hold the answers to modern-day problems such as climate change, health, and medicine.

Sacred and Science Go Together

Beresford-Kroeger had an unusual childhood. She was orphaned at a young age and brought up by elderly relatives, who steeped her in old Irish traditions and knowledge.

Growing up she learned that trees are a natural pharmacy—this is something traditional cultures have always known about. Beresford-Kroeger further shares that if it were not for our indigenous cultures, we would not have retained any ancient knowledge about our forests, and we need to thank them for this.

It's her deep knowledge that drives this work, a knowledge where spirituality and science go hand in hand.

She says, "I do believe that sacred and science go together."

An Environmental Poem for This Age: *Call of the Forest*

In her documentary, *Call of the Forest*, Beresford-Kroeger goes to the most beautiful forests in the Northern hemisphere. "From the sacred sugi and cedar forests of Japan, the ancient Raheen Wood of Ireland, the walnut and redwood trees of America, to the great boreal forest of Canada, Beresford-Kroeger tells us the amazing stories behind the history and legacy of these ancient forests while also explaining the science of trees and the irreplaceable roles they play in protecting and feeding the planet."

This is Beresford-Kroeger's call to action. She urges us to notice trees, to protect them, and to plant them—one tree a year for the next six years.

Her filmmaker says that "the tree is our perfect stepping stone back to nature. From the single tree outside your door to a vast forest beyond our view or conception, Diana believes the necessary re-engagement of person and tree is where real understanding of nature can grow from."

~*Questions*

When and where do you pick up the scent of these aerosols?

Chapter 15:
Elder Courchene: The Science and The Spirit

Mother Earth says, 'I bring you love'. This is not a sound we hear in our heads but in our hearts—it is universal.

—Elder Dave Courchene—Nii Gaani Aki Inini (Leading Earth Man), founder of Turtle Lodge on Sagkeeng First Nation.

Elder Dave Courchene shares ancient knowledge with us on how to reconnect to Mother Earth and listen to what she's telling us. He says that Mother Earth talks to us through the winds, the birds, the trees. She is alive and asks us to talk to the trees and to the water. Courchene says anyone can do this and asks us to give thanks to the trees, the water, and Creation.

"As humanity, we all need to learn this one simple, basic truth: That the earth is a living entity. She's alive. If Mother Earth did not have a spirit of life, then how can we have life?" he writes.

After reading Diana Beresford-Kroeger's work, I drew in the deep scent of balsam fir, jack pine, and spruce with new awareness, with new love for life. The work of this woman inspired me to go to traditional indigenous ceremonies at Turtle Lodge in Sagkeeng next to my hometown of Pine Falls.

The spiritual elder, Dave Courchene, is poetic in his prayers to the Creator as he tells us all the story of how we are meant to be guardians of the earth, trees, sky, fish, animals, and each other. These, Courchene tells us, are sacred laws of nature for all.

We listen and feel a part of the natural world around us. The young drummers start as the next part of the ceremony begins. This indigenous community already knows the secret of the forests.

> *The hills are alive with the sound of music,*
> *with songs they have sung for a thousand years.*
>
> —The Sound of Music

∾Questions

Keep a list of things you plan to say to a tree.

CHAPTER 16:
WILLIAMS: NATURE FIX

Scientists are looking with renewed interest at how nature affects our brains and bodies. Building on advances in neuroscience and psychology, they've begun to quantify what once seemed divine and mysterious. These measurements—of everything from stress hormones to heart rate to brain waves to protein markers—indicate that when we spend time in green space, 'there is something profound going on'.

> —Investigative journalist Florence Williams, author of *The Nature Fix: Why Nature Makes Us Happier, Healthier, and More Creative*

As my journey for answers continued, I found the research on green space and mindset empowering, scientifically riveting, exciting, and practical. I could see and feel the connection between my time spent around trees and my mindset.

I was now going outside every day, and my general condition visibly improved.

But I wasn't satisfied. I needed to find a reliable journalist who had a driving interest in trees/green space research. I needed someone who had talked with researchers about their work and findings. I needed someone to humanize these scientists for me.

Enter Florence Williams. She was spreading the word on the benefits of Nature. I listened to her TED talk, read her articles in *Outside Magazine*, and now wanted to grab a hold of a book.

Williams published *The Nature Fix: Why Nature Makes Us Happier, Healthier, and More Creative* in 2017. In this book she uses plain language to provide the stories behind nature research and researchers. Williams spent time with green space scientists around the world, including Japan, the UK, and Finland.

Forest Bathing in Japan

I had read about the "shinrin yoku" research conducted in Japan and wanted to get some context around it.

To me, at least initially, the entire concept, usually translated as "forest bathing," sounded like a slightly erotic hippie idea. It was not that at all.

As it turned out, the true meaning of "shinrin yoku" got lost in translation, and what we have in English does not actually capture the scientific rigor of the practice.

Right on track though, Williams went to Japan to meet a small number of physicians certified in Forest Medicine who "quantify nature's role in lowering stress and boosting mental health."

There she learned that in order to gauge human physiological responses to trees and nature proximity the Japanese researchers tracked changes in blood pressure, pulse, variable heart rate, salivary cortisol, and hemoglobin in the brain's prefrontal cortex.

Williams shares that Japan has 48 official forest therapy trails designated for "shinrin yoku" by Japan's Forestry Agency. To further their research, the Agency has invested about $4 million in the forest bathing initiative since 2003. Visitors who are eager to test this healing method are often asked to have their blood pressure taken to add to the data set.

Williams met with Dr. Qing Li, the father of forest bathing. Dr. Li is a medical doctor with a specialty in immunology earned from the Department of Environment Medicine at Nippon Medical School in Tokyo.

Dr. Li's primary interest when he started his research involved nature's effects on mood states and stress as manifested in the immune system. Specifically, he studied natural killer (NK) immune cells which can protect us from disease and can be measured in the lab.

Factors like stress and aging have been proven to reduce NK count. So, Li wondered, if trees did reduce stress, could they also increase NK count? The answer was a sound yes.

The Health Secret of Tree Aerosols

Li suspected that the aromatic volatile substances, or nice tree scents we breathe in when near trees, hold the answer. These are terpenes and other essential oils given off by evergreens and many other kinds of trees. Combined, these are sometimes called phytoncides. Scientists identified over 100 different phytoncides in the Japanese countryside. No tree aerosols were identified in the cities.

> *The health secret of trees seems to lie in the natural oils that are part of a plant's defense system against bacteria, insects, and fungi. Exposure to these substances can have measurable health benefits for humans. Physiological stress is reduced, for example, and both blood pressure and heart rate are lowered.*
>
> *Evergreens—pine, cedar, spruce, and conifers—are the largest producers of phytoncides, so walking in an evergreen forest seems to have the greatest health benefits.*
>
> —Dr. Qing Li, Immunologist, Department of Environmental Medicine, Nippon, Medical School, Tokyo

Interestingly, while Li was doing his research on tree air in Japan, Canadian botanist Diana Beresford-Kroeger was writing books on the very same subject. The two finally met a few years ago at the set of Beresford-Kroeger's documentary *Call of the Forest*.

Author Florence Williams points us to Li's study in which he tested the tree aerosol theory. Dr. Li enlisted 13 subjects whom he took to a hotel for three nights. In some of the rooms he used a humidifier to vaporize stem oil from the hinoki cypress trees. The cypress sleepers had 20% increase in NK cells. The same group reported feeling less fatigued in the mornings.

To Williams, Dr. Li stated that he himself uses a humidifier with cypress oil every night in the winter.

Williams says of her experience with Dr Li:

> *American researchers are mostly showing pictures of nature or sending people for loops around the campus green, the ones in Japan are pouring it into every orifice.*

Williams writes with elegance and humor. In the following, she tells us why tree aerosols work on us in an instant:

> *The role of the nose is a thruway to the brain. That is why some medications are administered nasally. Molecules of a certain size enter through the nose, bypass the blood-brain barrier and march right into the gray matter.*
>
> —Florence Williams in *The Nature Fix*

It is no wonder then that when we smell woodsy scents our mood lifts in a nano second.

Take Your Vacations in Natural Areas

Williams asked Li what else he would recommend. He simply said:

> *If you have time for a vacation do not go to a city. Go to a natural area. Try to go one weekend per month. Visit a park at least once a week. Gardening is good. On urban walks try to walk under trees, not across fields. Go to a quiet place. Near water is also good.*

Measuring Emotions and Mood States in the Forest

Wherever there are trees, we are healthier and happier.

—Dr. Li

In 2018 (after the publication of *The Nature Fix* in 2017), Dr. Qing Li published his own book, *The Japanese Art and Science of Shinrin-Yoku Forest Bathing: How Trees Can Help You Find Health and Happiness*, in which he asks us to notice how we feel before and after we spend time near trees.

He also led a study, "Emotional, Restorative and Vitalizing Effects of Forest and Urban environments at four sites in Japan." With 45 participants he used a Profile of Mood States questionnaire to measure their mood before and after being in a forest environment compared to an urban environment. The results showed that only the forest participants had feelings of vigor and recovery after the experience.

To measure mood, Li used an established psychological well-being scale, where emotions are quantified by intensity and fall into mood state categories.

Some of the emotions are: tense, angry, worn-out, unhappy, lively, confused, sad, active, energized, grumpy, drained, forgetful, and uneasy.

The mood states are: anxiety, depression, anger, vigor, fatigue, and confusion.

Mood Study Results

Only the forest bathers had feelings of vigor and stress recovery. The urban participants did not.

While other studies have shown that walking outdoors reduces depression, anxiety, and anger, Li found that only the experience of walking in a forest improved people's vigor and reduced fatigue.

Finland: You Need Five Hours a Month Outside

After her encounter with Dr. Li, Williams met with scientist Liisa Tyrväinen who runs the research division at the Natural Resources Institute of Finland. Tyrväinen felt the Japanese studies were too small. She wanted to run larger studies and see if the results would be the same.

Like Dr. Li, she used the Profile of Mood States, but her study involved 3000 city dwellers. The team asked the interviewees about their emotional and restorative experiences in nature. Tyrväinen obtained the same results Li observed in his smaller well being studies.

Her work also included a Restorative outcome scale with statements like:

— I feel calm
— I feel focused and alert
— I got several ideas

Based on these studies, Finnish scientists recommend spending at least five hours in nature per month. Five hours is the bottommost limit of time you need to spend in nature to gain the benefit of feeling restored.

A UK Economist Shows Place Matters Most in Terms of Our Happiness

Florence Williams knew that there was something good going on in the UK as well. She signed up to be part of an experiment run through the University of Sussex. Professor George MacKerron, an economist, led the study. He wanted to know if place mattered in terms of happiness.

MacKerron's research included one million geolocations. These places were loaded on a smart phone app with 2000 volunteer users. He factored in the vacation effect and looked at what made people happiest.

MacKerron's happiness variables results, as quoted in *The Nature Fix*, showed that:

— "We are least happy at work or being sick in bed, and happiest with friends or lovers."

— "The biggest variable, it turned out, was not who you are with or what you are doing—but where you are."
— "People are significantly and substantially happier outdoors in all green or natural habitat."

Something Big Going on in Scotland: National Initiatives

Staying with the UK, Williams wrote that academic Scotland had a new National Walking Strategy, and that access to green space nature had become a new national indicator for health.

Williams also reported that the Scottish government was underwriting a program called *Branching Out* to provide mental healthcare in outside environments. It involved spending three hours per week, for a duration of 12 weeks, in a woodland program. The results for people who had already tried the program showed reduced symptoms of depression and increased sociability, physical exercise, and self-esteem.

This was big and Williams knew it. She published her book before Scotland announced that its doctors were now legally allowed to prescribe walks in nature as medication—particularly for those aging with chronic disease (more in subsequent chapters).

Mitchell and Self-Esteem

Green exercise, that is, any physical activity performed outdoors (from a stroll in the park to a bike ride through the forest), lifts mood and self-esteem.

—Professor Richard Mitchell, an epidemiologist and geographer, and Co-Director of The Centre for Research on Environment, Society, and Health at the University of Glasgow, Scotland

Around the time I was pouring over William's book, I was discovering the research of Professor Richard Mitchell at the Institute of Health and Well-Being, University of Glasgow. Professor Mitchell studies self-esteem and mood in green places. His studies show that any activity performed in green space lifts mood and self-esteem.

Mitchell's study of 2000 participants found that "there was a 50% improvement in people's health if they were active outside around trees."

His work showed that activities done outside, in green areas, were 50% more effective in lifting mood and self-esteem than the same exercise performed in a gym.

Dr. Mitchell clearly didn't expect those results. He explains:

I wasn't surprised by the findings that exercise in natural environments is good for your mental health, but I was surprised by just how much better it is for your mental health to exercise in a green place like a forest, than in other places like the gym.

Smyth: How We Feel About Ourselves and Illness

In daily life, low self-esteem predicted more stress severity and symptom severity. And the opposite was also true. Higher self-esteem acted as a buffer in chronic illness.

—Professor Joshua Smyth at the University of Syracuse, Department of Psychology

Self-esteem is the way we feel about ourselves. Professor Joshua Smyth showed that our self-esteem affects our disease symptoms. In his study, 97 people with asthma and 31 with rheumatoid arthritis were asked five times a day for one week about how they felt. Smyth found that symptoms like pain and shortness of breath were greater in those with low self-esteem.

Taylor: We Are Fractal and So Is Nature

Taylor (…) is working with medical researchers to see if it is possible to restore brain function. He is showing stroke patients fractal patterns.

—Florence Williams in *The Nature Fix*, on Richard Taylor, Physicist, University of Oregon.

Reading *The Nature Fix,* Williams was the first person to introduce me to a concept I had never heard before: fractals. Like me, you may not have heard about fractals.

Fractals are repeating, branching patterns that make up our lungs, kidneys, heart beats, flowers, tree branches, clouds—and more. So, we are fractal and so is nature. When we look at fractals in nature, we are looking at ourselves. The eye and the body connect and respond.

> *I lead an interdisciplinary research network that investigates the positive physiological changes that occur when people look at fractal patterns. The experiments—which use eye tracking equipment to examine how people look at the patterns, and EEG and MRI probing techniques to quantify resulting brain activity—indicate that people are hard-wired to respond to a specific form of fractal found in nature, one that reduces stress levels up to 60%. This stress reduction is triggered by a physiological resonance that occurs when the fractal structure matches that of the fractal image being viewed.*

> — Richard Taylor, Professor of Physics, Psychology and Art; Head of Physics Department, University of Oregon

Taylor calls this immediate connection fractal fluency. When describing how fractal fluency takes place, Taylor says we do not have to stare at a fractal. We can get the same effect by walking down a hallway with windows or working by a window.

Taylor, The Artist

Early in his art career, Taylor had been studying Jackson Pollock's paintings and knew that there was something curious about them. Especially fascinating was the story of how a dejected and lost Jackson Pollock showed his friend how he paints. Basically, Pollock took a can of paint and, at regular intervals, splattered it on the canvas. He did this day after day on the same canvas, in the same way.

In an interview for Williams, Taylor shared that the more he looked at fractal patterns, the more he thought of Pollock's paintings and curiosity lead him to measure their electrical currents. Understandably, Taylor proceeded to analyze those patterns with the help of a computer, comparing them to forests. He found that the two patterns were exactly the same. In his published study Taylor says, "Pollock painted nature's fractals twenty-five years ahead of their scientific discovery."

Brain Waves, Blood Flow, and Our Emotions

Continuing with his studies, Taylor measured people's brain waves while they were viewing geometrical fractal images. After looking at the image for just one minute, the frontal lobes of the brain started producing alpha waves of a relaxed state.

Taylor used functional MRI to find out where the blood flow (thus attention) went when his participants looked at fractals and found that fractals engage the parahippocampus. This is the part of the brain involved in regulating our emotions.

Taylor has been using artificial fractal-based implants to restore sight to the blind. He says that "If you don't build fractal fluency into a bionic eye, not only have you lost the ability to navigate, you've also lost that symbiotic relationship with nature's fractal patterns."

Fractal Geometry

Fractal science and nature come together in the 1970's work of the mathematician Benoit Mandelbrot. He wrote the book *Fractal Geometry in Nature,* where he explained the visual side of nature through math formulas.

So, there you have it, fractal complexity is in nature, us, art, and mathematics. Taylor calls fractals "nature's trademark," because we need natural patterns to look at; they are a natural stress reliever to the busy, overwhelmed mind.

Time Outside Can Be Your Bio-Inspiration

In his interview with Williams, Taylor said he was using fractal fluency as "bio inspiration."

So, although fractal fluency is a completely new way of looking at the world, the basics of it have always been here, around us. The stress reducing feat of fractals, along with the mood elevating effect of tree aerosols combine to create powerful outside therapy. Let time outside become your bio-inspiration.

Sound Triggers a Startle Reaction in Our Sympathetic Nervous System

Perhaps because Florence Williams was struggling with her move from quiet Colorado to a home under a flight path in Washington, DC, her book also provides the results of her research on sound.

In *The Nature Fix*, Williams shares studies that say our brain reacts dramatically to sound. The researchers that Williams spoke to confirmed that whether asleep or awake, sound triggers a startle reaction in our sympathetic nervous system and elevates our heart rate, our blood pressure, and our breathing. We never get used to non-natural sounds, and the biological effects get worse over time.

Williams notes that there are few remaining quiet places in the world. As an interesting aside, she mentions that Gordon Hempton, a sound engineer based in Washington, DC, is traveling the United States in search of the few quiet places that remain.

We Don't Realize How Much Nature Elevates Us

Williams also says that "We think of nature as a luxury, not a necessity. We don't realize how much it elevates us."

While doing her research, Williams spoke with psychologist Elizabeth Nisbet at Trent University in Ontario, Canada. For a study, Nisbet sent 150 students either outside to walk along a path by the canal or through underground, well-used tunnels that lead to campus buildings. Before they left the classroom, she asked them to fill out surveys on how happy they thought they would feel on their walks.

It turned out the students consistently underestimated how much they would enjoy the outdoors and overestimated how happy they would be on the underground tunnel walk.

Florence Williams' Simple Coda: Go Outside, Often, Sometimes in Wild Places

As an English literature major, Williams often quotes Annie Dillard, Thoreau, Emerson, and other great writers throughout her book. While writing *The Nature Fix,* she visited one of her old professors, who impacted her way of thinking. Summarizing his themes, she says, "nature does everything to prepare you, to make you immune, or to gentle the shock. He doesn't say there is no shock."

This is Williams' simple coda:

"Go outside, often, sometimes in wild places. Bring friends or not. Breathe."

Use this as your personal coda.

The Science

By that time I was using this research to quell my deepest fears of dying too early, of stress leading to dementia, and losing control of my chronic disease. The research was speaking right to me and my needs. I had taken a sharp left turn from conventional medicine and healthcare. The answers lay in these deep interdisciplinary connections.

I started to feel very good about myself the more I went outside. And now I knew precisely why. My lifted mood and self-esteem affected my rheumatoid arthritis pain. I had less pain. All the time. When I looked into the branches of a tree,

I knew exactly what was happening in my eyes and then my brain. And it felt good. Very good.

And although I loved feeling good again, I felt positively great because I knew that by decreasing my stress with time spent outside, I was preventing future cognitive decline. I knew that once I went back to writing after being outside, I would be able to pay attention. I would be restored. I would learn new things and figure out new ways to solve my problems.

I knew that when I was taking my deepest breath of the day outside, I was breathing in medicinal aerosols. Anti-inflammatories and antibiotics topped my list.

Like investigative journalist Florence Williams, I wanted to share this profound outdoor science. Specifically, I wanted those in my demographic to know we have the most to gain from this research. And we are running out of time to implement it. The clock is ticking.

I have always loved radio and now was listening to podcasts. I started listening to Joanna Penn's podcast, *The Creative Penn*. Her smiling, lyrical British accent voice became my friend. She shared her world of independent book publishing, and I realized I had to sign up for her course, "How to Write Non-Fiction." Joanna Penn gave me something new to learn or to think about every day.

Florence Williams, Diana Beresford-Kroeger, Dr. Li, Professors Bratman and Berman lead the way for me. Joanna Penn shows me how to get the word out.

Next Stop: London, Visiting My Son and the Trees

Around this time, one of my sons moved to London, England. Naturally, my other son and I planned a visit. Since a lot of the best tree research comes out of the UK, we incorporated significant tree time in our activities.

We walked among the 170,000 trees in London's Royal Parks, also known as London's lungs. We wandered, strolled, and laughed through all eight of them and learned that London is one of the greenest cities in the world.

Like old buildings, ancient trees are a valued part of London's past. Trees are the very fabric of the culture. And everyone I met sounded like Joanna Penn.

∾ Questions

Do you seek out green spaces when on vacations?

If you have a garden, how much time do you spend in it?

Do you spend time in other green spaces?

Do you notice changes in your mood before and after going outside (e.g., any signs of feeling restored or energized)?

How do you feel about yourself (your self-esteem) before and after you go outside?

Do you notice a connection between your stress levels and how you feel about yourself?

Try to track your stress levels and your illness symptom levels five times a day.

How do you feel after you look into the branches of a tree (or other fractals). Can you think of fractals as your bio-inspiration?

Do you have a quiet space to visit outside?

Do you have a book that inspires you to go outside?

CHAPTER 17:
WE ARE ALL
UNDER HOUSE ARREST

Do you remember, as a child, going outside and playing all day? It is as if somehow our culture has moved to the inside. All the attractions and work seem to be going on there. How do we take back our habit of going outside?

According to the Canadian Human Activity Pattern Survey (CHAPS), we spend an average of 93% of our time indoors. This breaks down into two subcategories:

— 87% enclosed in buildings—working, on our phones, cooking, cleaning, and looking after loved ones, and
— 6% in vehicles.

These proportions are fairly constant across the various regions of the U.S. and Canada.

This means we spend only 7% of our time outdoors, or an average of 1.7 hours a day. I doubt that most of us even spend that much time outside every day.

Maximum security prisoners spend 2 hours outside each day. That is more than we get most days. It seems our indoor culture is under a kind of house arrest.

What Would 10% Outside Look Like?

If we wanted to increase our outdoor exposure to 10% that would mean an extra five hours a week outside.

In the 1990's, the U.S. Environmental Protection Agency (EPA) sponsored a study, the National Human Activity Pattern Survey (NHAPS), which involved 9386 people of all ages across 48 states.

The purpose of the NHAPS was measuring the effect of indoor cigarette smoke as the key indoor pollutant—in the 90's people were still smoking inside buildings.

How They Did It

In order to accumulate enough data, the agency measured human activity inside and outside by time and location.

NHAPS was conducted on a daily basis from late September 1992 through September 1994 by the University of Maryland's Survey Research Center.

Since then, smokers have moved outside, which is better for them and those around them. Now we need some kind of cultural rule to get us all outside more often.

Author Annie Dillard, in her book *The Writing Life*, sums up how we spend our days:

> *How we spend our days is, of course, how we spend our lives. What we do with this hour, and that one, is what we are doing. A schedule defends from chaos and whim. It is a net for catching days. It is a scaffolding on which a worker can stand and labor with both hands at sections of time. A schedule is a mock-up of reason and order—willed, faked, and so brought into being; it is a peace and a haven set into the wreck of time; it is a lifeboat on which you find yourself, decades later, still living.*

Feeling Beautiful Outside

The more time I spent outside, the better I felt. My website, TreesMendUs.com, was up and running. I was writing weekly blog posts about the health benefits of spending time near trees. I was feeling productive and happy. Readers were interested in the research.

After a while, I noticed that my face looked relaxed in my blog videos taken outside in the woods near my home. My voice was even calmer—smoother. I smiled more often. This worked like an instant facelift. There is something about the beauty out there, and the trees standing tall, that makes me want to do the same.

All of this was happening around the time beauty entrepreneur, visionary, and risk taker Jennifer Walsh joined my Facebook group where we encourage each other to get outside every day. It is called "Ditch Inside for Outside."

Walsh says, "What inspires me most is nature. Central Park is where I feel most inspired." I started to follow Jennifer's daily Instagram story. She is busy but always finds time to take a break and go outside. She posts her Central Park walk in the trees most days and inspires me to go on a stroll in nature. I can tell by her voice that she is happiest out there.

∽Questions

Do you have people who inspire you to go outside? Do you follow someone like Florence Williams or Jennifer Walsh, or a Facebook group to inspire you to go outside?

How much time do you spend out of doors each day? Or on the weekends? Track your outside episodes and time intervals during the day.

Can you list what keeps you inside?

Can you track when you consciously try to get outside (even for a few minutes)?

Can you shift your schedule around to get more outside time?

CHAPTER 18:
LANGER: NOTICE NEW THINGS

Noticing new things is what we do outside. As Ellen Langer points out, by noticing we become engaged; we become excited and our neurons fire. Noticing gives us new energy.

Langer's research has also discovered that the mind is very powerful in helping us to be healthier, happier, and to live longer. Her work fits with the research on awe.

> *Pretend you are travelling and focus on seeing the new in things you think you already know.*
>
> *Simply noticing the new in the old accelerates the inner work of freeing your mind from negative thoughts.*
>
> —Ellen Langer, award-winning social psychologist, Harvard University.

No Big Solution: It Is Easy and Fun

What I love about Langer's mindfulness is that it is not meditation. It is something different. It is more direct, immediate, and simple. It is all about noticing new things. That's it.

"It's a lot like opening up to see all the different shades of green in a tree." Langer is also an artist, and noticing the many shades of green in a tree put the start to her noticing studies.

Langer says that when we notice new things, our neurons are firing—we are energized. The nice thing about it is that it is so easy.

Freezing Our Understanding of Aging and Disease Is Deadly

Langer, now in her 70's, is turning her attention to those who are aging with chronic disease. She says we are used to taking a word or two of something and thinking we know the entire concept. We believe that things are stable and predictable.

She shares that the deadliest approach we can take about aging and disease is to "freeze our understanding" about anything. As a scientist, she wants us to keep a mindset of uncertainty because things can be understood in many ways. Langer wants us to see "the power of possibility."

Medical Diagnoses and Our Desperate Desire for Certainty

When speaking of our medical diagnoses, Langer says that our "desperate desire for certainty makes us miss the opportunity of fully tapping into the power of uncertainty."

She states that we like to create categories and then get trapped by them. Disease categories are an excellent example of the concept of fixed thinking, she notes.

Langer asks us to tap into our mindset of "universal uncertainty." She does not mean individual uncertainty of self-doubt; we have to look at the bigger picture:

"I don't know, you don't know—what is going to happen. This allows you to help each other."

Instead of Focusing on What You Think You Know About Your Condition

> *Instead of focusing on what you think you know about your condition, stop and notice when it is better and when it is worse; when you feel pain and when you do not. Paying attention to change is good for you.*
>
> —Ellen Langer

In a 2019 interview Langer shares she is working with people who have chronic disease. She eagerly explains that most people living with stress, for example, think they suffer all the time. For her study on the topic, her team of researchers contact participants at random times of the day and ask, "How do you feel now? Is it better or worse? Why do you feel better now?" Then many solutions become obvious, says Langer.

Langer is adamant that when you attend to changes in your symptoms, you recognize that you don't feel stressed, in pain, or ill all the time. Mindfulness changes your mind and body.

"Our world of concrete facts keeps us thinking that what we know is a constant; that facts are absolutes. But it seems that our factual information is stopping us from seeing the nuances."

Langer does not apply her work to specifically being outside in green space, but we can. Simply stopping and noticing, as Langer shows us, will immediately put us in the present.

Hold Off on Worry

> *Don't throw your emotions at it again... Why pay twice?*
>
> —Ellen Langer

Langer advises, "no worry before it's time." Worry is about something we might do tomorrow, but today we can say to ourselves, "Everything I do today I am going to enjoy."

She asks us to make things fun, and notes that anything can be fun if we have this perspective.

Returning Control to Patients

We may have a chronic condition, but we are capable of noticing when we feel fine and when we do not. Everything is changing all the time.

—Ellen Langer

In her course of work, Langer is also investigating time perception, blood sugar variations, and vision test results. Her researchers speed up or slow down time, change medical results, and then measure participants' responses. In every case, the perceived test results are what matter not the real results and time.

As Langer says, "If we think we got more sleep, we feel more rested. If we think our blood sugar will go up, it does. If we think we are able to see less letters on the eye chart, that's what happens."

And, it logically follows that if, as in my case, I was told that sunshine will negatively impact my health, I was afraid to go out and enjoy the sun.

With her work on symptom variability, Langer's aim is to return control to the patients.

The Antidote to Worry, Anger, and Confusion

Langer's suggestion is to simply ask ourselves:
"Is this true? Do I need to panic? How do I know things will turn out this way?"

According to Langer, the antidote to worry, fear, anger, and confusion seems to lie in these four questions:
— How is this a good thing?
— How is it a bad thing?
— How do I even know it is going to happen?
— If the worst does happen, what are the advantages?

Ellen Langer's mindfulness doesn't ask us to deny our experiences and pretend that everything is wonderful.

Rather, at the end of these questions, "the thought that had captured you, to which you had previously been only reactive, now you can look at and be responsive if you want. But you are back in the driver's seat. Not the thought."

In a recent interview with Krista Tippet, Langer said that when something happens, which we don't like, we should ask ourselves, "Is this a tragedy or an inconvenience?"

Our Beliefs Are the Only Things That Matter

Langer says our mindset is a belief that orients the way we handle situations—the way we sort out what is going on in our lives and what we should do about it. She explains that most people go through life mindlessly, but we could have a richer life with mindful living. She says: "Our beliefs are the only things that matter." Through years of research, Langer has figured out how to get better results later in life by slightly shifting our mindset.

What the Mind Believes, Our Body Delivers

All of Langer's studies show that "what our mind believes, our body delivers."

To illustrate her words, Langer ran a fun study which showed that our biological age is what it is, but our mental age and capacities could be those of a much younger person if we just shift our mindset.

Challenge Our Thinking Around Age

In her landmark Counterclockwise Study of 1979, Langer showed the impressive power of human mindset. For the experiment, she enlisted men in their 70's and 80's to live for a week as though it were 1959. Then she took the group for a week-long stay in a monastery which had been retrofitted to a time 20 years prior.

The men were to live there for a week as if the past was the present. So, playing the part, they spoke about past events as if they were just happening in their current life. Half of the men were told to pretend they were literally back in the 50's and live like they had at the time; the other half were just told to reminisce.

A set of cognitive and physical tests was conducted both prior to and following the week-long stay. And at the end of the experiment all participants had improved their results. Curiously, the ones who had pretended to be young had improved the most.

In their thoughts, those men had gone back in time to when they had looked and felt younger. At 50 they had been in their prime, they had been in charge. Their minds and bodies had been more vital. In letting themselves go back in time they had truly believed that they were those people again—and it had worked. They had begun to look younger, stand taller, have better vision, hearing, and cognitive function.

During the study, the men had seemed to grow younger. Even the test results had confirmed that height, weight, posture, vision, hearing, and IQ had all improved. Mentally putting themselves back into their youth had actually made their bodies rewind!

Altering the Way We Think About Ourselves

Langer believes that by "altering the way we think about ourselves and our worlds, we can actually bring about change in our bodies and lives."

According to Langer, the Counterclockwise Study shows "how we can actively challenge these ingrained behaviors by making subtle changes in our everyday lives."

Mindlessness in the Medical World

In an interview Langer shared that her personal issues with her grandmother's and her mother's breast cancer led her to take a "closer look at the mindlessness almost inherent in the medical world."

She also discussed a study she ran in the early 70's where her team went to a nursing home and gave people a plant to take care of. Langer says:

"When you take care of a plant you notice the way it changes, when it needs water… so we encouraged this mindfulness. The comparison group were just given tender love and care (and nothing to notice or be mindful of)."

When the team went back to the nursing home 18 months later, they found that there were twice as many people alive in the mindful group (the ones noticing their plants) compared to those making no decisions.

Langer concludes: "So there I had these very striking findings on how it is just thinking these thoughts that leads to longer life and also to happiness."

Talk to Your Mind

Remember that your brain is continually calibrating. Many of your thoughts are not true. You don't have to listen to the ones you don't like. You can stop paying attention to them.

You can talk to your mind. You can tell it that you don't know how things will turn out. You can tell your mind that there might be opportunity in the circumstance. You can let unhealthy thoughts drop. The moment you step outside you will let go of everything.

As soon as you get outside into green space, your muscles will relax, your breathing and heart rate will slow down on their own. I honestly know no other way to get this kind of instant peace. As soon as you go outside your uneasy thoughts drop away. Your exhaustion will give way to a sense of awe. You will be able to see the light in the trees, in yourself, and in others.

∽Questions

Let's apply Ellen Langer's mindset tools.

The moment you step outside, can you notice one new thing? (This exercise is as effective as meditation—it places you in the present). Pretend you are a tourist.

Do you have a plant, garden, or tree to take care of (e.g., noticing when it needs water)?

Does going outside slightly shift the way you think about yourself and your world (helping you to live longer)?

If you get test results that you don't like, can you avoid throwing your emotions at those results? As Langer says, "why pay twice?"

If you worry about upcoming test results or doctor's appointments, can you use Langer's "hold off on worry" approach to help you? E.g., "What is going to happen? I don't know. You don't know. So let's help each other."

Even on very ordinary days at home, "can you say to yourself, everything I do today I am going to enjoy?"

Make a list of the things you will hold off on worrying about now.

If you worry about feeling worse or your chronic disease progressing—noticing how you feel at the moment is good for you. Ask yourself at various times of the day:

— How do I feel now?
— Is it better or worse?
— Why do I feel better now?

Are there aspects of your illness that you can see you can have more control over now (pain, sleep, stress)?

When you are outside, are you more fun? Do you take yourself less seriously? Are you less afraid?

Are you more in control of your emotions when you notice something new?

When something that you don't like happens to you, ask yourself: Is this a tragedy or an inconvenience? Keep track.

CHAPTER 19:
KELTNER: AWE

When we are filled with the sight of nature then we can begin to think of things outside of ourselves.

> —Keltner, Professor at Berkeley, University of California, Director of Greater Good Science Centre

According to Keltner, there are important evolutionary reasons for awe in response to nature. It's good for our minds, bodies, and social connections.

Five separate studies showed similar results, namely, that awe, "an emotional response to something that transcends our frame of reference," has immediate health benefits.

His research shows that awe makes us pause, the body quiets down so we can take in the information.

Awe makes us slow down and stop worrying. It makes us feel more generous, more humble, happier, and healthier. Awe also sharpens our thinking. It transforms negative feelings into positive ones.

The same researchers also observed that awe is triggered by simple things like gazing up into the branches of trees. And awe inspired by noticing a green forest can give perspective and help readjust your view on the meaningful things in life.

How They Did It

In one experiment, Keltner's colleague Paul Piff used a grove of eucalyptus trees near Berkeley. He staged a small accident to see if awe influenced kindness.

"Participants first either looked up into the tall trees for one minute—long enough for them to report being filled with awe—or oriented 90 degrees away to look up at the facade of a large science building," reported the study.

They then met a person who stumbled, dropping a handful of pens into the dirt. Sure enough, the participants who had been gazing up at the awe-inspiring trees picked up more pens. Experiencing awe seemed to make them more inclined to help someone in need. They also reported feeling less entitled and self-important, unlike the other study participants.

In further studies, Keltner and his team found that awe made people more modest, less narcissistic, and kinder toward others. The researchers summarized that awe happens as little bursts of wonder.

～Questions

When and where have you felt a positive emotional connection to nature?

Are there moments that inspire you when you are in green space?

When you notice a new thing, do you become engaged and excited (your neurons are firing)? Does noticing give you new energy? Try to remember the moments outside that you felt energized today and write them down.

When you are outside, do you get little bursts of wonder and awe? Does this make you slow down and stop worrying? List the things that you stopped worrying about today.

CHAPTER 20:
I WISH I HAD KNOWN

I've been soaking in this research for the past couple of years. Now, I wish I had known all of this information the minute I was diagnosed with chronic disease. I wish I had read about it years before too. Right after my divorce would have been perfect timing. That was almost 20 years ago.

Now my wishes are for you.

If you are afraid of dying too early, I hope you know that:
— Being around trees makes you live longer. (James, Crouse)
— Noticing new things (outside) helps you to live longer. (Langer)
— Being in green space makes you have less disease, makes you happier, feel richer, and live longer. (Berman)
— Just thinking these thoughts can lead to a longer life and happiness. What our minds believe, our bodies deliver (Langer)

If you have fears about anything, and especially getting sicker or older, I hope you know that:
— A few minutes outside, close to trees, will effortlessly flip your mindset to positive. (Bratman)

— Your brain is continually calibrating. Many of your thoughts are not true. You don't have to listen to the ones you do not like. You can stop paying attention to them. You can let unhealthy thoughts drop.
— Your outside mindset allows you to look at what parts of your identity work for you and which ones do not. This is adaptive self -reflection. (Nolen-Hoeksema)
— This outside mindset perspective allows you to reframe your life and edit the thoughts that do not help you.
— Patterns in nature do more than reduce our stress levels by 60% to relax and comfort us. (Taylor) They also make us pause, slow down, stop worrying, amaze us, and fill us with little bursts of wonder or awe. (Keltner)

If you have low moods and self-esteem, I hope you know that:
— After being outside for 5 minutes, your mood and self-esteem will soar. (Mitchell)
— And that higher self-esteem predicts less stress severity and less symptom severity. Higher self esteem makes you less susceptible to stress. (Smyth)
— We all underestimate how much change is ahead of us, and how things are constantly changing all of the time. Higher self-esteem makes you less susceptible to stress.

If you think you need to meditate but have no energy, I hope you know that:
— The minute you step outside your nervous system automatically switches from sympathetic (fight/flight) to parasympathetic (rest and digest). Your breathing and heart rate will slow. This instantly regulates your emotions.
— You simply have to get outside, and your body will do the rest. When you have lots of parasympathetic activity, your stress levels improve— you can regulate your fear and anxiety emotions. (Van den Berg, Brown)

If you are afraid of disfiguring loss that may come with chronic disease or aging, I hope you know that:
— You will feel your happiest outside; (MacKerron) that you will love life and yourself again. (Barton, Pretty)
— You simply have to notice something new to be in the present. (Langer)
— By taking action (going or looking outside, taking care of a plant inside) you are changing the way you think. (Langer)

If you are afraid of losing your memory or your ability to concentrate (brain fog), I hope you know that:
— The stress reduction part of your brain is growing every time you go outside. (Kuhn) This helps you to cope with stress more easily, so you won't drain your brain power.
— By spending time outside you are improving your short-term and long term memory. By spending time in green space you are decreasing your stress levels. Lower stress in time spent in green spaces restores your ability to pay attention, to learn new things, and to problem solve. (Berman, Bratman, Barton, Brown). This restoration of attention (and other cognitive skills) prevents possible dementia. (Scott et al)
— Your brain is always growing and adapting at any age. Spending time close to urban or suburban trees can change your brain structure. By simply practicing the outside habit, you are buffering (or immunizing) yourself against future stress. You are developing stress resilience. (Ulrich) You are decreasing your chances of cognitive decline and dementia.

If you are hiding inside, I hope you know that:
— We all spend, on average, 93% of our time inside. (National Human Activity Pattern Study) Start small to develop your habit of visiting trees, shrubs, and grass around you.

— The mere action of going outside changes your thoughts and the way your body responds to illness and stress. Trees and nature will help you mentally and physically. All you have to do is get there. (Dr Li)

If you are holding your breath in chronic sadness, I hope you know that:
— Breathing in tree air is a powerful non-pharmaceutical prescription. By breathing outside, you are inhaling directly into your lungs a natural pharmacy of bioactive tree aerosols. These contain anti-inflammatories, antibiotics, antivirals, and antiseptics. (Diana Beresford-Kroeger, Dr. Li)

If you cannot get outside, I hope you know that:
— You simply have to look outside into the branches of a tree (or at an image of nature) to set your body to a calm state. (Ulrich, Van den Berg)

If you are losing your ability to be employed, I hope you know that:
— When you go outside near trees you will feel more alive, new energy filling every part of you. It will become easier for you to focus. You will have more ideas and new vigor. You will figure it out. Everything will fit together again. (Dr. Li)

If you become agitated by your age or the extent of your diagnosis, I hope you know that:
— What your mind believes—your body will deliver. By altering the way you think about yourself and your world you can actually bring about change in your body and life. (Langer)

If you want to know where to start to fix your worries about aging with chronic disease, I hope you know that:
— Mindfulness is built in the moment we step outside. Noticing is what we do outside. Once we are in green

space we can see that things can be understood in many ways. In our desperate desire for certainty (eg disease categories) we take a few words of something and think we know the rest. In this, we miss the opportunity of uncertainty. Use the phrase "I don't know and you don't know how this is going to go, so let's help each other." (Langer)

If you are too busy to go outside, I hope you know that:
— You are happiest when you are outside. (MacKerron) It is not who you are with or what you are doing that is the biggest variable in your happiness—it is where you are.
— Brief interactions with nature will disrupt old patterns of thinking and allow you to imagine new possibilities. (Bratman, Berman, Langer, Van den Berg)

If you are feeling overwhelmed, I hope you know that:
— Being outside allows you to change your world—and mindset. Instantly. Once the outside environment takes away your negative thoughts, you will be able to pay attention, to learn, and to problem solve. (Bratman, Berman, Van den Berg)
— You can have control. You can notice how certain behaviors affect you; for instance: I am fine now that I am outside. I am not so fine when I have been sitting at the computer for an hour.
— You can find solutions to your disease symptoms that do not involve medical intervention. Solutions that can better your state right away. (Langer) You can believe in other solutions to aging with chronic disease. You can look outside and go outside to find them.
— You can say to yourself, "Yes, my test results can be troubling, but most of the time, and particularly when I am outside, I feel healthy, happy, and beautiful. My body is doing what my mind is telling it to do." (Langer)

If you think you are no longer beautiful, I hope you know that:
— When you are outside, your face relaxes and you smile more easily. Your winkles soften, your face lifts, and your eyes sparkle.
— When you are outside, your self-esteem and mood lift. This makes it easier to stand up taller and take in the world. Notice a new spring in your step as you invite others to enjoy this outside moment with you. Emotions are contagious.
— When you pretend you are travelling you see things that you think you already know in a new way. You become engaged, excited, and your neurons are firing. (Langer)
— Going outside takes away your fears and helps you to be gentler to yourself and others.

If you think all you can put in your brain are facts about aging with chronic disease, I hope you know that:
— Going outside makes you aware of your thought processes.
— As you notice new things outside, you deepen your knowledge of trees and nature. This is good for you and yours. As you are drawn into something beautiful or interesting, they will join you. Together you can focus on something "other."
— Kimmerer says she shows her children how to love gardening so that they will know, after she is gone, that the trees and plants will always be there to care for and watch over them.
— An outside mindset changes the way you see yourself and your world around you. Your outside mindset has the power to edit your thoughts and to reframe your identity.
— Instead of focusing on what you think you know about your condition, stop and notice when it is better and when it is worse. Paying attention to yourself and your thoughts is good for you.

— Wherever there are trees, by spending time near them you will live longer, prevent dementia, and control your chronic illness.
— You are already there, you already have these solutions. You just have to see it, know it, and practice it.

Spending time in green space is free—but takes awareness and practice. The next section, "Ways of Being Outside," will give you some ideas of how others use the outside as their procedure for well-being and for living longer.

PART 3:
WAYS OF BEING
OUTSIDE

Chapter 21:
Scientists Who Go Wide:
Kimmerer and Haskell

> *Listen to the songs of plants to pay deep attention, so we can fall in love with the world again.*

> —Robin Kimmerer, author and Professor in Environmental and Forest Biology, State University of New York College

There are few scientists who write about their quiet relationship with nature; Robin Kimmerer and David George Haskell are among them.

Kimmerer is an indigenous botanist. Her open perspective to being outside helped her to figure out what to do out there.

If, at first, you are not sure what you should be doing when you go outside, Kimmerer advises to let that feeling go.

A Professor of Environmental and Forest Biology at the State University of New York College of Environmental Science and Forestry, Kimmerer combines her heritage with her scientific passions.

An indigenous elder once said to Kimmerer, "The best way to find something is not to go looking for it." This, Kimmerer admits, is a hard concept for a scientist, such as herself, to accept. But she is the first to tell you to "watch out of the corner of your eye, be open to possibility."

An Intimate and Emotional Connection

Kimmerer gently reminds us that as adults we often shed the curiosity of nature. We need to reclaim that deep attention that kids pay to plants.

According to Kimmerer, science puts "the polish on our ability to see things clearly through intense attention." But we need other lenses too. We need a more gentle and equitable approach, like the indigenous "two-eyed seeing" that allows for a bigger perspective which includes the intimate and the emotional lenses.

Kimmerer notes:

> *Just as you can pick out the voice of a loved one in the tumult of a noisy room, or spot your child's smile in a sea of faces, intimate connection allows recognition in an all-too-often anonymous world. This sense of connection arises from a special kind of discrimination, a search image that comes from a long time spent looking and listening. Intimacy gives us a different way of seeing, when visual acuity is not enough.*

We need to see plants as living beings, Kimmerer points out in her writings. Rather than treating plants as inanimate "it" objects, we should give them a name that makes sense to us. She gives mosses names that make sense to her—green velvet, curly top, and red stem. She also uses their scientific Latin names.

Kimmerer, along with Langer, believes in noticing something old in a new way:

> *You notice something that was always there but now you see it with a surge of expansion and sudden clarity. That experience is both humbling and joyful.*

This is how she expresses her observations in writing:

There is an ancient conversation going on between mosses and rocks, poetry to be sure. About light and shadow and the drift of continents. This is what has been called the 'dialect of moss on stone'—an interface of immensity and minuteness, of past and present, softness and hardness, stillness and vibrancy, yin and yang.

A Year-Long Watch of a Patch of Forest

Science deepens our intimacy with the world. But there is a danger in an exclusively scientific way of thinking. The forest is turned into a diagram; animals become mere mechanisms; nature's workings become clever graphs.

> —David George Haskell, author and Professor of Biology at the University of the South in Tennessee.

Haskell shows us how to look at nature with a careful and empathetic eye. He writes beautifully about his time spent in the same one square meter land in the Tennessee forest near his home.

Almost daily, he sat, listened, focused on his breathing, and observed a little patch of forest. He performed no research. He took to the forest with a magnifying glass, binoculars, and a notebook—"and of course, my senses."

Haskell writes lyrically about the seasons during this one complete year of visiting his patch of forest. This is how he talks about the changing fall forest floor:

The sound of my footsteps changed radically this week. Two days ago, the forest floor was deep with sun-dried fallen leaves. Silent movement was impossible; walking was like traversing a field of crinkle wrap. Today the crash and crunch of the autumn's shed leaves are gone. Rain has relaxed the tense curls, and animals move across the wetted, muted ground with silent steps.

～Questions

Have you noticed something outside that might make you fall in love with life again?

Do you go out in the forest or green space looking for something in particular? If not, what have you discovered outside recently?

Do you give plants and trees your own names? Would you like to?

Is there a square of forest or green space that you can visit each week? Note some possible places you'd like to observe.

Would you be interested in following Haskell's approach of writing short essays/posts to learn and reflect on your place?

CHAPTER 22:
WRITERS WITH CHRONIC ILLNESS

Thoreau: Living Beautifully with Chronic Illness

In short, all good things are wild and free.

— Henry David Thoreau

Most of us know Henry David Thoreau, who lived in the 1800s, as an essayist, poet, philosopher, teacher, and naturalist. We don't think of him as the symbol for the open, outside-loving mindset that is perfect for living well with chronic disease.

But that he is, and today, Thoreau has become a totem of returning to nature.

Henry David Thoreau died of tuberculosis at the young age of 45, after decades of living a thoughtful and beautiful life spent in the outside world.

According to his biography, Thoreau's parents were the ones who taught him to love nature. In his early life, he spent most of his time outside, learning about "every bug, bird, berry, beast, every fruit, and every flower."

Tuberculosis, a plague at the time, also claimed the lives of his grandfather, his father, his brother, and his older sister.

Thoreau became ill with his first bout of tuberculosis in his 20s. He became so weak and exhausted that he couldn't return to his studies at Harvard.

"The mass of men lead lives of quiet desperation," Thoreau once wrote in his later years. He lived with his chronic illness for decades.

Outside Was His Lifeline

Thoreau knew the secret ingredient to staying well and alive was the outdoors' restorative power. So, he was active outside for hours at a time. Every day.

To restore his health, he immersed himself in nature. For decades he lived well with tuberculosis. Over a hundred years ago, Thoreau knew that getting outside was his lifeline. He said:

> I think that I cannot preserve my health and spirits unless I spend four hours a day at least—and it is commonly more than that—sauntering through the woods and over the hills and fields, absolutely free from all worldly engagements.

He could not bear to be inside, probably because he only felt well when he was among nature. His words show that Thoreau had empathy for those who have no choice but to stay inside:

> When sometimes I am reminded that the mechanics and shopkeepers stay in their shops not only all the forenoon, but all the afternoon too, sitting with crossed legs, so many of them—as if the legs were made to sit upon, and not to stand or walk upon—I think that they deserve some credit for not having all committed suicide long ago.

Thoreau knew he had to move. He knew that being in nature was saving him: mentally and physically.

He frequently wrote about his day-to-day close-up encounters and observations of nature. His many works show his great attention to detail in the world outside.

Thoreau's Sister's Support

Henry's sister, Sophia Thoreau, looked after him as he became very ill and fell victim to tuberculosis. She was a teacher and a naturalist, who loved to garden and cultivated her own flowers.

According to an article published by the *Thoreau Society*, Sophia Thoreau's drawing of the cabin by the pond is on the cover page of *Walden; or, Life in the Woods.* The cabin is "nestled among the evergreens and lacy deciduous trees." This simple sketch "has become a symbol of individuality and self-reliance throughout the world."

He Did Not Travel Far

Thoreau lived simply. He did not travel to faraway places, probably because he did not have the energy or the money for it. Nonetheless, he stepped out of his door every day and walked for hours, determined to see the exotic in the local.

His writings clearly show that Thoreau enjoyed his daily walks that were to him, each day, different.

My vicinity affords many good walks; and though for so many years I have walked almost every day, and sometimes for several days together, I have not yet exhausted them. An absolutely new prospect is a great happiness, and I can still get this any afternoon. Two- or three-hours' walking will carry me to as strange a country as I expect ever to see. A single farmhouse which I had not seen before is sometimes as good as the dominions of the King of Dahomey. There is in fact a sort of harmony discoverable between the capabilities of the landscape within a circle of ten miles' radius, or the limits of an afternoon walk, and the threescore years and ten of human life. It will never become quite familiar to you.

Not only did Thoreau find new discoveries on his everyday walks, but he found adventure too:

> *The walking of which I speak has nothing in it akin to taking exercise, as it is called, as the sick take medicine at stated hours—as the Swinging of dumb-bells or chairs; but is itself the enterprise and adventure of the day.*

Henry Thoreau's active lifestyle and love of the outdoors helped him live with tuberculosis for decades. Isn't it time to think of Thoreau as having the new outside mindset that we need for aging beautifully with chronic illness?

Jarem Sawatsky: Finding a Healing Way

Jarem Sawatsky, a former professor, is a Manitoba native who has Huntington's Disease. His 2017 book *Dancing with Elephants: Mindfulness Training for Those Living with Dementia, Chronic Illness or an Aging Brain* is about finding a healing way to face the terminal disease.

In his book, Sawatsky notes that he doesn't discuss "the kind of healing that takes away the disease but the kind of healing that opens the heart to love." He calls this dancing with elephants because "dancing is a way of engaging with what we fear the most."

There is a section in his book where he talks about walking and asks these questions:

> *Why do we have to go to the other side of the world to find sacred spaces? Such luxury is for the rich and able-bodied. If we cannot touch and respond to each step around and outside of our home, what makes us think we will do better in another place? If we do better in another place, will it make us mindful of the sacred when we return?*

Sawatsky made the decision to walk close to home. He called this activity "walking meditation" and "urban pilgrimage" and approached it in a Ghandi type of way: no electronics and no wallet. His goal was to walk all the streets in Winnipeg, and he almost did it before the -40 below zero winter freeze took hold.

He summarizes his walking experience thus: "This was a beautiful time for me. I saw parts of Winnipeg that I had never seen."

With these words, Sawatsky reminds us that walking outside is a simple practice. It is a way to celebrate life in the face of relentless loss.

∼Questions

Are you, or someone you know living with terminal illness?

Although you may be on the same walk every day, do you notice different things each time?

Do you go out in the forest or green space looking for something in particular? If not, what are your recent outside discoveries?

CHAPTER 23:
DOCTORS IN SCOTLAND
PRESCRIBING NATURE

When I was researching the mental health benefits of time spent near trees, I realized I had to dig deep to find what I was looking for. Fortunately, the scientific research was there, and it was solid, but strangely, my physicians and many other specialists had never heard of it.

I was determined to know why and raised the topic of trees and health with my physicians. Uncomfortable silence followed. It felt to me that it would take decades for the medical establishment in Canada to pay attention to this body of evidence.

However, while I was writing this book, physicians in Scotland started prescribing time in nature to patients with chronic illness. Through the Prescribing Nature Project, nurses and doctors explain and promote to patients the many physical and mental health benefits of spending time outdoors. The project's main health focus is on people with chronic disease.

So, it seems Scotland is way ahead of the game, sponsoring tree research and accommodating a national health indicator for distance to green space from home address.

"The physical and mental benefits of connecting with nature have been very well evidenced by numerous studies," says Makena Lohr, a spokeswoman for the Centre for Sustainable Healthcare in Oxford. "It's high time that the healthcare sector became aware of that. Those who don't live in Shetland do not have to miss the health benefits either."

The Prescribing Nature Project is run by The National Health Service in Shetland, Glasgow, and The Royal Society for the Protection of Birds, Scotland. The RSPB helpfully created a calendar resource for patients that provides outdoor ideas and activities largely focused around birding.

The project leads expect this bold initiative to deliver improved outcomes for those with chronic illness. Its aim is to help people to manage their chronic conditions more easily.

One of the lead physicians in the Nature Prescription Project is clear about why she supports this idea.

"I want to take part because the project provides a structured way for patients to access nature as part of a non-drug approach to health problems," states GP Chloe Evans from Scalloway Health Centre, who oversaw the pilot program. "The benefits to patients are that it is free, easily accessible, allows increased connection with surroundings which hopefully leads to improved physical and mental health for individuals."

At the moment, 10 health clinics across Shetland prescribe nature to their patients. The plans are to extend the project to more areas and health boards in the UK.

Already, the program has grabbed headlines around the world. Let's find ways to get the information into the hands of our physicians.

In the meantime, we don't need a doctor's prescription to get outside. Here's to your open outside mindset!

ᗅ Questions

Can you write your own prescription for an outside mindset? Name your medicine as "outside green space" or "tree time."

The required duration of time is: X minutes/hours of time spent outside. The frequency is: how often you need to go outside.

Here's an example:

Take 30 minutes of tree time x 5 days a week.

Or:

Tree time: 30 minutes x 5 days/week.

Practice writing out your outside prescriptions yourself or ask a loved one to do it for you. E.g., Look outside into grass and trees 5x/day for 5 minutes.

You can have several on the go. No risk of side effects or adverse drug interactions.

CHAPTER 24:
DOSES OF TREE TIME

Greenspace Dose—Response

As a result of countless studies, researchers are increasingly treating exposure to trees like we currently treat drugs. Time spent close to trees (dose) shows large health benefits (response).

The following section "microbursts of nature" explains that your "dose" may be 3 minutes in greenspace and your "response" to greenspace will be stress reduction. What if you have been under stress for some time?

Microbursts of Nature

In the previous sections you read about how prolonged stress affects your ability to pay attention and keep track of the tasks at hand. The research also shows that stress over the long term speeds up the loss of brain power (cognitive function). This increases our chances of short- and long-term memory loss and dementia. Managing stress is not just about feeling better in the moment, it is about protecting ourselves from losing mental capacity.

Stress in these studies is defined as fear and anxiety. It is based in unhappy childhood, ongoing strains, major life events, and daily difficulties.

Unconstructive thought patterns, or negative rumination, shows up as stress. When we concentrate on past stressful events, we are overthinking. By doing this we are overusing our cognitive resources or brain power. This drains the brain power we have left over for non-stressful times.

Scientific studies show the immediate effect of quick bursts of nature as:

— Looking out the window or at images of nature relieves stress in minutes and also eases future stress.
  • To prove this, Ulrich used EEG of brain waves to show that higher alpha brain waves were associated with relaxation and serotonin production. In the 1970's and 80's, he used heart rate and pulse rate transit time (time it takes for the heart rate to change) and found that heart rate slowed minutes after looking at a nature image.
  • In 2013, Vandenburg showed that after 5 minutes of exposure to nature or nature images one can recover from stress and even accumulate a buffer to future stress.
  • Even spending only 1–5 minutes outside can lift self-esteem and mood. (Mitchell, Barton, Pretty, Daniels)
— Taking micro breaks to go to a garden, a back yard, a park, or a forest lowers your stress levels. Research (McKerron) shows that "people are significantly and substantially happier outdoors in green or natural habitat."
— Step outside for 1–5 minutes and you will notice your body's response. (Dr. Qing Li) It's as easy as paying attention to how you feel before and after you go outside. (Profile of Mood States, Grove, University of Western Australia)

Dr. Li's Tips (of Forest Bathing Fame)

Dr. Qing Li gives these tips for forest bathing:
— Go out into the green space around your home and community.
— Go out in your garden or sit under a tree.
— Walk to your destinations (shops, school, gym, work).
— Walk under trees whenever possible.
— Breathe deeply when you are near trees. Exercise outside whenever possible.

If you have time for a vacation, do not go to a city. Go to a natural area. Try to go one weekend per month.

Visit a park at least once a week. Gardening is good. On urban walks try to walk under trees, not across fields. Go to a quiet place. Near water is also good.

—Dr. Qing Li

Finnish Tips About Time Required in Green Space

In Williams' *The Nature Fix,* she shares that the Finnish government research team asked 3000 city dwellers about their emotional and restorative experiences in green spaces (Tryvainen).

Word choices included:
— I feel calm
— I feel focused and alert
— I got several ideas

According to research findings, cortisol (stress hormone) levels drop even in city parks with pavement and some street noise. Just 15 to 45 minutes are enough to improve mood, vitality, and feelings of restoration.

One published study Williams mentions showed that "5 hours a month is the lowest amount of time to get the effect, then after if you go for 10 hours, you will reach a new level of feeling better and better."

According to Williams' calculations, this means:

5 hours a month = a couple of times a week for 30 minutes
10 hours a month = 5 days a week for 30 minutes

~*Questions*

Are you ready to log your outside time? Chances are you already have outside habits. Maybe you go outside to feed the birds or tend a plant.

Regardless of your reasons, keep track of the time you spend outside over the days, years, and across seasons. Then log your observations in a journal. Bring your log outside to track your progress. This data collection will help you to break down going outside into small steps.

Start your entries like this:

How do I feel *before* going outside?
Tired? Ok? Weary? Fine? Energized?
Date:
Duration:
Location:
How do I feel *after* being outside?
Energized? More ideas? Better able to concentrate?

CHAPTER 25:
HOW TO NOTICE THE OUTSIDE

Our internal landscape is a near perfect reflection of the external world. No wonder looking at fractal patterns can reduce stress as much as 60%. (Taylor) When we look at fractals, our neurons fire in new ways and our minds open.

Think of the way a tree grows. One trunk divides into two branches, which split into two more, and on it goes.

Notice the natural patterns in nature, and you will begin to see them everywhere: tree branches, the veins in tree leaves, the cracks in the ground, snowflakes, cloud formations, flower petals, layers of leaves on the ground, rivers, lakes, seashells, stones, acorns, and so it goes.

Our brains' neural pathways are trained to do a "search image" process, looking for complex visual patterns in a particular configuration. "Then the synapses fire and the stars come out," says Kimmerer.

Slow down. Draw close to see those patterns in nature emerging before your eyes. Get to know the fractal geometry of individual tree branches, a snow flake, a perfect pebble, an acorn, the clouds.

Think not of what you see but what it took to make the endless repetition of patterns. Look at how these patterns replicate in new growth. Notice the architecture of the forest. Make the landscape even more of a marvel.

Take Your Deepest Breath of the Day When You Are Outside

One deep breath flips your nervous system from anxious (sympathetic) to calm (parasympathetic). When you are outside you are breathing in aerosols that will make you live longer and feel richer, happier, and healthier.

Tip: Breathe in for 7 seconds; hold it in; then release for 5 seconds, concentrating on your belly.

Give a Tree a Name That Has Meaning to You

Stretch your language to include new things that you notice. When you are outside things become clear, bright, and distinct again.

Be surprised by the beauty of the natural world, of the human heart and mind. Having words for these things helps to make them more compelling and clearer.

Every nuance of tree architecture has a word—and speaks of careful observation.

> *Give a tree its own name. You don't have to say, that is an oak. You can see it as an individual. Your words give them life.*
>
> —Kimmerer

Below is my list of things to notice. When I pay attention to them, I have elevated moments, inspired moments, and transcendent ones. Be excited if you pass no one. Notice the moment that you are alone in this spectacularly beautiful place.

Smile widely and notice:
  — that different trees have different scents
  — the smell of the soil
  — the scent of rain

— the deep wooded fragrance of pine and fir
— other scents in the forest
— the breeze on your skin
— the movement in the tree branches
— the sounds that each tree makes
— the different sounds that oak leaves, pine boughs, and poplar leaves make in the breeze
— how you are feeling
— birdsong
— the warmth of the grass in the sunshine
— how a tree sways in the wind
— how the bark of a tree feels when you run your hand over it
— the motion of leaves in the trees
— the soothing sounds that leaves make in the breeze
— the green light and shadow of a tree
— the old and the new in this place
— the calls filling the night at the start of spring
— crows calling overhead
— the voices of the rain
— the warmth still lingering in a rock
— every bird you see
— dense grey fog clinging to the trees
— the pointy spires of spruce trees as the fog covers and uncovers them
— how the sunlight hits the river or lake, creating sparkles or a mirrored glass reflection.

Be inspired to experience some sights and sounds from Lorna Crozier's poem "The Wild In You":

A Winter's Sleep: so much sleeping in this place. Think of all that lies beneath the snow.

Anne Lamott, in her work *Bird by Bird*, quotes Gary Snyder:

Ripples on the surface of the water—where silver salmon passing under—different from the ripples caused by breezes.

CHAPTER 26:
THINGS TO DO OUTSIDE

Before you look at my list of things to do outside, remember there is always a small step you can take. There is always a point where you can be successful.

The suggestions below are accessible to all of us. Going outside is free. Let the outside open your mind in a new way today. Know that your heart rate will slow down and your breathing will deepen when you step outside. These are changes that we cannot fake. They just happen when we look or step out.

When You Are Inside Looking Out

1) Make a list of places you would like to check outside.
2) Keep a window list of birds you have seen.
3) Make a list of the trees around your home or office.

Your Approach to Going Outside

Be like Thoreau who believed going outside was the adventure of the day. And although you may be in the same area, notice something different each time you are out there. Thoreau, perhaps because he was not well, learned the value of staying put. He committed to his sense of place. Get familiar with your neck of the woods. Define yourself as a placed person.

1) Go outside whatever the weather. Feel the exhilaration of the wind, snow, or rain on your face.
2) If you are in a new city, use Google Street View because it shows how green the city is at street level. Plan your route.
3) Bend down and touch a plant for a few seconds.
4) Brush your fingertips over the moss.
5) Pick a tree to observe. Take photos of it over the year to see how it changes in each season.
6) Find a perfect pebble.
7) Look for an intact shell of a lake clam.
8) Tend some plants.
9) Walk with poles (easier on the joints and provides more stability).
10) Go biking.
11) Listen to birdsong.
12) Breathe in the sound of trees and birds.
13) Close your eyes and listen to the rain.
14) Hear the motion of leaves in the trees.
15) Put a magnifying glass in your backpack. Check the size and shape of anything interesting, like moss.
16) Use a pair of upside-down binoculars as a microscope.
17) Feel the cushy matt of moss.
18) Pick up a rock. Imagine where it might have come from. What forces shaped it? Was it deposited by glaciers? Part of an old riverbed? Wet the rock to see its colors.
19) Learn the names of rocks. Count the layers in a sedimentary rock.
20) Hum. When you hum you breathe deeply. Humming or any self-created sound increases the oxygen level in your cells.
21) Plant some bulbs.
22) Use a tree app to identify trees.
23) Pick two different kinds of grasses and really look at them.
24) Make a meal using the flower of a dandelion.

25) Watch pollinators at work: butterflies and bees.
26) Follow a bee or a butterfly.
27) Listen to and copy the sound of a tree. Talk to the tree. Thank it for all it does for you.
28) Notice that spruce have round needles and balsam have flat needles.
29) Draw a snowflake.
30) Write your thoughts and insights about nature in your Outside Mindset Companion Workbook.
31) Look for tracks and signs of animals.
32) Watch a crow for courting behavior (flipping in the air).
33) Pick up garbage in the woods or on the beach.
34) Notice tree colors—the many shades of green and brown.
35) Make or get a wind sock to appreciate the speed of the wind.
36) Welcome the birds home from the south with a celebration.
37) Join a club that goes outside.
38) Borrow a dog and take it for a walk or play games.
39) Make pictures on the beach using seaweed, sand, and rock. Let the waves wash them away.
40) Stand looking over a river bank or a cliff top listening to the sounds of the water, trees, and birds.
41) Touch the water in a river or lake.
42) Spot a tree and find out more about it. What type of birds does it attract?
43) Use a sheet or towel to capture the wind.
44) Find the hairiest lichen within a mile radius.
45) Find a tree with fruit—feel its texture.
46) Find a bud on a tree—feel its texture.
47) Turn over some soil and plant some flowering plants.
48) Take a tree minute—step outside to look at a tree.
49) Take a bird minute—step outside to hear the call of a bird.
50) Spot birds returning from the south.
51) Visit the nearest UNESCO site near you.

52) Bury your face in the grass.
53) Make a daisy chain.
54) Have a gardening routine.
55) Grow fresh vegetables.
56) Plant a tree.
57) Go to a botanical garden.
58) Listen for a bird and then try to spot it.
59) Find a place outside to sit and be still. Notice how you feel.
60) Turn over a rock and see what is there.
61) Don't mow the lawn—and watch the bees and the birds move in.
62) Carve out some time for yourself to go somewhere you have never gone before.
63) Visit nature trails around you. Discover rare and local plant species. Breathe in the smells and sounds.
64) Sit on the ground or on a rock and listen to the sound of the breeze in the trees, to the creaking in tree trunks, to the birds.
65) What is your favorite sound of the season? Go listen for it.
66) Take your hood down.
67) Go for a walk on the beach when the water is low. Notice the ripple fractal patterns in the sand; look for clams.
68) Listen at a distance to waves, wind, trees, birds.
69) Make a meal outside.
70) Watch the waves.
71) Clouds are described as wispy (cirrus), fluffy (cumulus), and layered (stratus). What clouds are in your sky today?
72) Look at a tree trunk for woodpecker holes, birds' nests, types of fungi growing on trunks and branches.
73) Write an email to a special tree that you admire: "I know you probably get told this all the time, but the way your branches reach up to the sky makes my heart soar."

74) Kick through a pile of leaves. Notice the rustle and crunch.

75) Take part in a local walk to support your lake or forest.

76) Notice the different types of moss under your feet.

77) Appreciate a cloud.

78) Help a neighbor with their garden.

79) Write a worry on a stone and throw it into the lake, river, or sea.

80) Get close to a tree and smell it (re-wild your senses).

81) Find 10 different species of trees and mosses in your area. Take photos of them all.

82) Look for fish jumping in a lake.

83) Listen for the sound of frogs. Record them on your phone.

84) Create a rock sculpture on the beach.

85) Feed the birds in your yard.

86) Do you know a balsam from a spruce tree? Look back on your year and see how far you have come.

87) Find a good place to breathe in tree aerosols (somewhere quiet too).

88) Walk into the wind.

89) Listen for the different sounds leaves make. Oak leaves flap. Poplar leaves flutter in the slightest breeze.

90) Go pelican watching.

91) Explore some sand dunes in your area.

92) Go outside to be with the phases of the moon. Try to look at the moon through some trees.

93) Try to see a pickerel (or any fish) disappearing into the shadows.

94) Follow a path in the woods.

95) Listen to and copy a birdsong—try talking to the bird.

96) Listen to live or recorded birdsong for 5 minutes a day.

97) Listen to and copy the sound of a tree—try talking to it.

98) Make a sound map. Place an x in the centre of the page and then illustrate the sounds you hear around you.

99) Notice what time of day the light sparkles on the water.
100) Notice the patterns of light and darkness in the shadows of a tree.
101) Notice how the ground feels underfoot today (soft, wet, quiet, or crinkly).
102) Breathe in to the count of 7, release to the 5. Feel it in your tummy.
103) When you breathe in the woods you are inhaling a cocktail of health promoting bioactive substances that trees, shrubs, plants, and the soil release into the air.
104) Join a volunteer cross-country ski club.
105) Put a rock that you have collected from somewhere else into a new place that you love outside. Give it back to nature.
106) Notice big things, vast things, and little things up close.
107) Smile to yourself. Congratulate yourself for getting outside. Give yourself a high-five. Do a happy dance. Give yourself a hug or a pat on the back.

CHAPTER 27:
TREE ID

Trees gave me a sense of belonging, a sense of being away, and a new perspective on my life with chronic illness. If you want to deepen your scientific knowledge of trees, you need to know what a tree is.

What Is a Tree?

Let's start with the definition. A tree is a woody plant with a single erect perennial trunk at least 3 inches in diameter at breast height (DBH).

Most trees have shaped crowns of foliage. Spruce tree tops are tall, narrow, and pointy. They look to me like a cluster of church spires.

A tree is over 13 feet tall.

A shrub is a small, low growing woody plant with lots of stems.

A vine is a woody plant that depends on something to grow on.

Make Up Your Own Name for a Tree

We don't often stop to interact with individual trees. Give a tree a name that means something to you.

Actress Judi Dench names her trees after each of her friends who have died.

In her film, *My Passion for Trees*, Dench listens with a stethoscope to the flow of sap in the maple trees on her property.

CHAPTER 28:
TREE ID APPS

A new tool in the GLOBE Observer app allows citizen scientists to take tree height measurements, information that can be compared with data from NASA missions.

Credits: NASA GLOBE Observer

The GLOBE Observer app provides a step-by-step guide for people to collect scientific data on their surroundings. With the new GLOBE Trees feature of the app, observers record tree height by tilting their phone up and down to align the screen with the tree's top branch and base, and pace off the distance to the tree; the app does the rest to calculate the tree's height.

"With the GLOBE Observer, everyone can become a citizen scientist and easily take measurements to better understand their local ecosystem," said Brian Campbell, GLOBE Trees science lead. Observers can measure one tree or hundreds. The data points—along with a GPS tag of the tree's location—are sent back to NASA and collected in a database. Anyone can visualize all of the tree height and other GLOBE data simply by visiting the GLOBE website.

Itree Is a Tree Mapping Tool

Canadian botanist Diana Beresford-Kroeger talks about tree aerosols drifting down from tree tops. For her film, *Call of the Forest*, she created a free Find A Tree App you can use to pinpoint your location on a map and see what trees grow in your temperature zone. This is how she explains the app on the film's website:

> One of the primary 'selling' features of the Find A Tree App is its flexibility.
>
> The app features a number of filtering options, which allow the user to narrow down the potential species in question to just those within the user's area.

In fact, users can narrow down the search criteria so much that the app effectively becomes, in the designer's words, the "Woody Plants of Where You Are Standing."

British Trees App

I also found a British tree identification app from the Woodland Trust, the conservation charity. This app offers facts, folklore, history, and uses of local trees. According to their website with this app you can:
   — "Recognise species in spring, summer, autumn or winter, even when there aren't any leaves on the trees.
   — Use the app when you're out and about—no internet connection needed.
   — Family friendly and easy-to-use.
   — Packed with detailed images and illustrations for accurate identification.
   — Read fascinating tree facts.
   — Add identified trees to your favourites.
   — Use the map to record trees you've found.
   — Share your saved trees with friends.

— Add your saved trees to the public map.
— Use the map to explore thousands of ancient trees nationwide."

LeafSnap

LeafSnap is another free app. Developed by a bunch of scientists with the Smithsonian, it only identifies trees of the northeastern United States.

In its nature, LeafSnap is an electronic collection of field guides meant to help users learn about trees. The app also allows you to take photos of trees which then get uploaded to a central database. After a short process, during which the system runs its recognition algorithm, it gives you a species identification.

Tree Finder

The online resource ThoughtCo. has a leaf key. It allows you to identify a tree by snapping a photo of a leaf or needle and uploading it in their simple finder. This tree finder is designed to help you identify most common North American trees. When you use the app, you can send your tree identification questions to "Dr. Dendro."

Google Street View

Another thing to do is use the Google Street view if you are in a new place. This shows how green a city is at street level. Then you can plan your treed route.

How to Identify Trees on Your Own

First, find out if a tree will or will not grow in your area. Trees have unique habitats and will not naturally grow where the climate doesn't suit them. You can usually eliminate trees that don't normally live wild in the forest where your tree lives.

For example, the coniferous (needle) forests of Canada and the Northern United States are mainly spruce, balsam, cedar, jack pine, and tamarack. The deciduous (leave) trees in these forests are poplar, birch, maple, and oak. Douglas fir grow in the Pacific Northwest and ponderosa pine in the forests of the Rockies.

Then identify trees by their parts. The tree parts, like leaves, fruit, bark, and overall shape, are unique to each species and can be used as identifiers.

Colors, textures, smells, and even taste will also help in finding the type of a particular tree.

Steps to Tree Identification

1) Collect a leaf or a needle and ponder the following:
    a) The presence of needles or leaves would help you identify a tree as coniferous or deciduous.
        i) Coniferous trees have pine cones and needles that stay on the tree all year long.
        ii) Deciduous trees usually have broad, flat leaves that fall off in the autumn.
    b) Note the type and color of the leaf or needle. Recognizing the leaf shape often is the easiest way to identify a tree.
        i) An oak leaf, for example, has deep lobes and rounded edges.
        ii) Pines have needles, and cedars have flat scales for leaves.
2) See if there are any fruit/nuts or flowers on the tree.
3) Study the bark of the tree for color, texture, and other characteristics.
    a) Some trees have unique bark, such as the paper birch. Its bark peels off in smooth, papery, curled sheets.
    b) Some trees have "eyes" where branches once were. For this reason, poplar trees are called "watchful trees."
4) Step back and notice the shape of the tree. A tree with drooping branches could be a weeping willow. Trees with pointy spire-like tops often turn out to be spruce.

Chapter 29:
Words That Work

With words at your disposal, you can see more clearly.
Finding the words is another step in learning to see.

—Kimmerer

These words will help you become consciously aware of your thinking around aging with a chronic disease, around going outside, and will, consequently, help you to unhinge your patterns of staying inside.

When things are happening in your life that you don't like, remember to step outside. You can use Ellen Langer's words for yourself: "Is this true? Do I need to panic? How do I know things will turn out this way?"

Langer says the antidote to worry, fear, anger, and confusion is held in these questions:

— How is this a good thing?
— How is it a bad thing?
— How do I even know it is going to happen?
— If the worst does happen, what are the opportunities?

Dr. Langer's mindfulness doesn't ask you to deny your experiences and pretend that everything is wonderful. She shows you how to take hold of your thoughts about what is happening. She gives you the language to take control back. This is true freedom.

Affirmations

On her podcast, *On Becoming Wise,* Krista Tippett writes, "The words we use shape how we understand ourselves, how we interpret the world, how we treat others. Words make worlds."

Having words you can call on when you have worries or anxieties running through your mind is another helpful thing to do. Often, people get attached to negative thoughts like, "I'm too old for this," or "This is going to be awful" or "My body is falling apart."

Many people find it helpful to have specific alternative words to focus on. Affirmations, that is, positive words, work on the prefrontal cortex. When you speak them out, they are like a mirror to your subconscious.

Negative thoughts like, "I will never get outside," "Why do I even try to be outside?" "I won't be able to do it," "Nothing helps," or, "I don't have the strength to go outside" make you feel weak.

If you step outside you can see these thoughts from a distance and replace them with more empowering thoughts that can help you create a different story for yourself.

Find some words or sentences that help you focus your mind in a positive way. Move from worry to hope. Use words that are personal to you and describe what you want to happen. You can say, "I am calm" even though you may not be quite there yet. Focus on trying to feel the words.

Below is a list of well-being statements from outside research studies. Use these affirmations when you feel you need them. Repeat the ones that speak to you—at least seven times a day and especially when worries creep in.

Create a different story for yourself by saying:
— Every day I have plenty of opportunities to go outside.
— I am okay when I am outside.
— I am fine right now.

— I am not so fine when…
— I can get outside, even if it is for a few minutes.
— I am peaceful and at ease when I am near trees.
— I am calm near trees.
— I love this tree.
— I have the strength to go outside.
— I let go of my worries/anxieties when I am outside.
— I am dealing with my worries/anxieties.
— I am in control of my worries/anxieties.
— My worries/anxieties are thoughts, not reality.
— I am letting go of all I cannot control.
— My body is working for me.
— I breathe in and out near trees.
— I feel better when I am outside.
— I am healthy and strong.
— I can and will go outside, and here is how…
— I am more than able to do this because…
— I feel beautiful when I am outside.
— Others are attracted to me when I am outside.
— When I am outside, I feel fine.
— When I am outside, I feel free.
— When I am outside, I forget I have a chronic disease.
— By allowing myself to be happy, I inspire others to be happy as well.
— Happiness is contagious, I spread happiness to others and absorb happiness from others.
— I can tap into endless happiness inside myself at any time.
— I find joy and pleasure in simply looking at a leaf.
— I have a deep and powerful love for the outside, trees, plants, and for other living beings.
— I enjoy what I see in others for exactly what they are— for their unique qualities.
— While outside I communicate openly with myself and with others. I smile and look for joy. I feel no conflict.
— I am completely myself when I am outside.

— I feel confident outside.
— Being outside helps me to want the best for those I love.
— I know that the people around me are doing the best they can—with what they know at the time.
— I constantly surround myself with those who love the outdoors—and who lift me higher.
— I know what I need to do when I am outside. Nature sparks learning in me.
— I can feel the energy in the trees and the plants. I am surrounded by tree energy.
— The more I notice, the more I am in the present.
— I give myself the gift of freedom from past losses.
— I keep an outside mindset of universal certainty. The world can be understood in many ways.
— I will move on in joy from this moment on.
— I choose outside wonder over inside worry.
— All is well in my life.
— Healthy tree, healthy me.
— The more engaged I am outside, the more I am in the present.
— I am safe. I am loved. This is now my natural state.

Take actions to support your thoughts.

Step outside for a one-minute bird break or go for a 30-minute stroll. In both cases, your mindset shifts instantly.

Stress leaves. Negative thoughts vanish. Happiness moves in. Your self-esteem soars. You have new energy.

Within seconds of getting outside, celebrate your success. According to Stanford University behavioral scientist B.J. Fogg, PhD, this will reinforce your new outside habit.

The second you get outside, say to yourself any of these quick things:

— You are awesome!
— Good for you!
— Bingo!
— Yay me!
— Good job!

— Wooooot!
— You've got this!
— Aha, not too shabby!
— We have a new plan, Stan.

or:

— Sing, "I feel good…do,do,do,do"
— or just sing your favourite happy song to yourself.
— Give yourself a high-five.
— Smile and pat yourself on the back.
— Give yourself a hug.
— Do a victory dance.
— Do a wonder woman stance.
— Click your tongue.
— Do hip thrusts.

After spending some time outside, you might say to yourself:

— My memory and concentration are improving right now.
— I feel happy right now.
— I feel good about myself right now.
— Aha! I am going to live longer now.
— I look good out here.
— I can move out here.
— When I breathe in out here, I am breathing in natural medicine.
— My breathing has slowed, my heart rate is going down, my body and mind are calm.
— I am breathing in to the count of 7, and out to the count of 5.
— I don't need a doctor's prescription for this.
— I am taking back control of my life.
— I am noticing new things, so I am living my life in the present.
— I am being mindful without meditating.
— Any dose of nature works.
— My body is working for me.

— I feel free.

— I love life again.

— I love me again.

Going outside to be near trees gives you the distance from your emotions. It gives you a new context to conceptualize and reframe your life in a positive direction.

Age Beautifully with an Outside Mindset

Going outside can dramatically improve your mood, memory, and energy level. Don't wait for your doctors to prescribe going outside. Change your life by changing your mindset. Save your time and money by going outside.

Live longer and be more relaxed than you have ever been. Feel beautiful instantly by stepping outside. Be free and happy. Don't worry ahead of time. Keep a mindset of universal uncertainty: "I don't know and you don't know."

Don't let the fixed disease category box you in. Notice something new outside. By doing this, decrease your stress instantly. Grasp the fact that you may be preventing memory loss or dementia by going outside. Breathe deeply outside near trees. Share the science of green space and trees with others who want to age beautifully.

Smile to yourself because you are living in the present by simply being outside. Your outside mindset is helping you age beautifully, despite your chronic illness.

As you age with chronic disease, you will become more energized and happier. You will become more vital and refresh your life. You will become more beautiful. Others will be more attracted to you. With your new outside mindset you will change the way you live, love, and breathe.

Do you need to feel better at this very moment?

Be Nice to Yourself: Go Outside

You don't have to wait for your next vacation or the weekend. Invite yourself outside to sit for a few minutes or for a short stroll.

Go outside. Get yourself out there. Go no matter how you feel. You don't have to wait. Go out in any kind of weather.

Going Outside: An Act of Self Compassion

Think of going outside as an act of self-compassion. Think of going outside as treating yourself with kindness and gentleness. Try treating yourself as you would treat a friend. Invite yourself outside for a walk.

The moment you step outside and notice one new thing you will be in the present moment. No need to meditate.

You May Not Be Aware of Your Own Mind State

You may not be aware of your own mind state. Your thoughts might be squirreling around in a constant mental chatter.

You might be suffering. You might be criticizing yourself. You might be in incredible pain. The stress hormone, cortisol, might be racing around in your veins. Your reptilian brain might be lit up. You might feel attacked. You might be completely unaware that these are thoughts—not you.

Going outside is a way to feel safe again. The science is clear. Our minds and bodies respond to trees, shrubs, and grass. Being out for a short time in any green space around trees turns down our stress response. Going outside changes our thought patterns—and lifts our mood.

It's Easier Than You Think

Going outside even for a few minutes will give you comfort. Start small. A minute or two a day will do the trick.

Since we all spend 93% of our time inside, going outside often, for microbreaks, will shift your mindset.

As a society, we have unlearned our ability to go outside. Our inside schedules have taken over. It is not easy to step away from our inside work, screens, beds, couches, food, and loved ones.

If you can see a tree, look into its branches. You are reaping the benefits of stress-reducing fractals.

Go outside for an optimal mindset. Once you are outside, call this your beautiful outside mindset.

A Compassionate and Easy Way to Help Yourself

Going outside is the compassionate way to deal with loss and frustration. This will be your way to embrace how difficult life can be. Let stepping outside be one sure way to help you through tough times.

Open Your Heart to Yourself

Going outside is a way of being open-hearted to yourself. It will help you to be open-hearted to others. You will know what to do. You will know what to say. Your stable sense of self will come back to you. You will trust yourself again.

Going outside will be your way to lift your spirits without the pitfalls of medication. Going outside will give you a pause to figure out what is going on in your body, mind, and heart. You will be able to create a plan for your life.

Be Curious About Yourself

Going outside is an act of self-awareness and self-compassion. It is like laying a hand over your heart in times of pain. It is noticing your body's cues.

Be curious about yourself. Before you go outside, ask yourself: How am I feeling? Pretend you are your close friend. When you go outside ask yourself: Where is my focus now?

These questions alone will put you in the present.

Use Going Outside as Your Self Care Protocol

You don't have to stay inside. Go outside with intention. Give yourself space. Give yourself attention. Change your brain chemistry. Use the outdoors to take away stress and help you to ease your emotions. Nourish your mind and body.

Start today. Very soon going outside will take care of itself. You won't have to wait for some future time to feel good outside. The comfort of the outdoors will be yours. You will be in charge of your emotions. Use the outdoors as your protocol to feel better again. Like your doctor who has protocols and guidelines for treating your illness, you will have yours too. Going outside will become your self-care protocol. You will develop your own outside guidelines.

Let the greenspace research take you to a new place. Take back your outside mindset. Reclaim the wonder and curiosity of outside green places. Increase your chances of living longer, prevent dementia, and control your chronic illness. Lift up your mood, boost your energy, and control your mindset. Set yourself free.

Conclusion

What we know from science is that those of us who are aging with chronic illness have the most to gain by going outside to green spaces often.

Two years ago, I was trying to get better by resting inside my house. I was miserable. The person I was back then does not exist anymore and my transformation into a happy outsider all stemmed from my decision to step outside. The outside research took me to a new place. It will do the same for you.

So, if you are still hesitating about feeling better as you age with or without chronic illness please take that first step outside. It will change your life.

Use this pneumonic to develop and keep your outside mindset:

CONTROL

You are now in CONTROL. You are in control of your emotions, your thoughts, your stress levels, your disease symptoms, and your life.

C is for Count the times that you step outside in a day. Every minute counts. Those who spend more time around green space live 12% longer than those who don't.

O is for Outside spaces. Remember your backyard, local park, and trees.

N is for Notice. Noticing puts us in the present immediately. No meditation required. Notice how you feel about yourself outside (self-esteem).

T is for health giving Tree aerosols. Say it with me "Trees Mend Us" and "Healthy Tree, Healthy Me."

R is for Respirations—note how they slow—breathe in through your nose, breathe out through your mouth. Your nose is a through way to your brain.

O is for Outstanding—congratulate yourself for getting outside. Talk to your brain. Tell it what is happening.

L is for Look at nature's fractal patterns. Reduce your stress through the eye-brain connection. L is also for loving your life again!

About Verla Fortier

Verla Fortier is a Nurse with a Master's Degree in Health Science. She has worked in Emergency, Intensive Care, Rehabilitation, and Community Health Nursing. Verla is a former Director of Surgery at The Toronto Hospitals and a retired Associate Professor of Nursing at McMaster University in Hamilton, Ontario. Since learning she has systemic lupus three years ago, she has been blogging at TreesMendUs.com. There she shares research of how spending time near trees makes you happier and healthier.

Connect with Verla

Website and blog: www.treesmendus.com
Twitter: TreesMendUs@verlafortier
Instagram: verla_fortier
Facebook: TreesMendUs
Youtube: Verla Fortier

NEED MORE HELP GETTING OUTSIDE MORE OFTEN?

This is a special invitation to put this book into practice, to change your behavior—and make your life better.

Sign up at www.TreesMendUs.com to get your FREE:

— "30-Day Outside Mindset Challenge" complete with your Outside Mindset CONTROL worksheet to keep you on track. The worksheet helps you to remember why you want an outside mindset, what to do and not to do, and what you will get out of this challenge.
— Facebook group "Ditch Inside for Outside." In this group we practice and figure out how to eliminate our own roadblocks to the "30-Day Outside Mindset Challenge."
— Outside Mindset meditation for you to listen to when inside or outside.
— List of my personal Outside Mindset affirmations that I use daily to boost my health and self-esteem.

Please Leave a Review

If you liked the book, please leave a review on Amazon.

It is critically important to get reviews on new books when they launch. Apart from helping persuade people to give a new writer a shot, reviews help drive early sales, which means Amazon takes notice and markets on my behalf.

In case you haven't previously left a review on Amazon, please do not be afraid to do it now. You can change your review at any time.

If you buy the book on Amazon you get a verified purchaser badge next to your review. This review carries great weight.

If you did not purchase the book on Amazon, you can still leave a review and it counts.

How to Leave a Review

1) Sign into your Amazon account. In the search bar type these keywords: Mindset, or Outside Mindset, or Live Longer.

2) Scroll down and find the place on the page titled "Review this product" and click "Write a customer review."

3) Select a star rating and leave an honest review. It is fine if it is short. If you use any of the words in the book's title, like Mindset, Outside, or Outside Mindset, this helps.

4) If you like other reviews of this book, please mark these as helpful. This helps me too by showing your engagement with other readers of the book.

5) You're done. And I thank you for your support. It means a lot. If you are not up to leaving a review, that is fine too. If I have helped you, then mission accomplished.

ACKNOWLEDGEMENTS

I have a lot of people to thank for this book. First and foremost, my sons, Max and Jesse Fortier, who have pulled for me each step of the way while I was writing my first book. They continue to delight and surprise with their young wisdom.

My parents, Tom and Edna Fortier, were with me as I wrote this book. I leaned on memories of their courage, intelligence, and humour in the face of my father's multiple sclerosis and then my mother's dementia. In choosing to discuss my parents' decline and death, I know that my sisters, Patty and Gail Fortier, may not necessarily have told their story the way I did. Nonetheless, my sisters helped me at every turn with shared warm memories of our parents.

Because I have drawn deeply on the major concepts in the work of scientists, I have many brilliant thinkers to thank. Professors Gregory Bratman, Marc Berman, Ellen Langer, Diana-Beresford Kroeger, it is an understatement to say your work has changed my life. Professors David Haskell, Robin Kimmerer, Richard Taylor, Richard Mitchell, Dan Crouse, Peter James, Stacey Scott, Simone Kuhn, Jo Barton, Daniel Brown, J. Pretty, Dacher Kelner, and Magdalena Van den Burg, you have all enriched my book. Investigative journalist Florence Williams, you led the way with your book *The Nature Fix: Why Nature Makes Us Happier, Healthier, and More Creative.*

The technical aspects of preparing the manuscript were carried out with great proficiency by Vanya Drumchiyska, who helped me to say what I wanted to say. She went through every draft with me meticulously.

Thank you to Jane Dixon at JD Design for the book cover and your professionalism.

My partner Phil Hallford has been a constant and encouraging force. Every idea in this book we have talked through together and, in many instances, also lived through together.

I am indebted to more than one hundred treesmendus.com subscribers who give me their time, tell me their stories, and let me into their lives. They are not mentioned in these pages. But they are all here just the same.

BIBLIOGRAPHY

"'Making Sense' Part 2, Professor Ellen Langer." YouTube video, 7:38. Posted by "Gandy Dancer Films," October 30, 2017. https://www.youtube.com/watch?v=ZinY1QTtplM/.

"Dr. Diane Hamilton interviews Ellen Langer." YouTube video, 25:22. Posted by "Diane Langer," February 22, 2019. https://www.youtube.com/watch?v=tfLpEh9nluc./

"Fractals: The Hidden Dimension." YouTube video, 15:01. Posted by "Darren Buckley," December 12, 2012. https://www.youtube.com/watch?v=xLgaoorsi9U./

"The Biological Effects of Sympathy, Gratitude, and Awe." YouTube video, 5:19. Posted by "World Economic Forum," February 21, 2018. https://www.youtube.com/watch?v=fmS8L6pQYss/.

Allen, Summer. "The Science of Awe: A white paper prepared for the John Templeton Foundation by the Greater Good Science Center at UC Berkeley." *Greater Good Science Center at UC of Berkeley*, 2018. https://ggsc.berkeley.edu/images/uploads/GGSC-JTF_White_Paper-Awe_FINAL.pdf/.

Anae. "Fractals in psychology and art." *Univesity of Oregon* (blog). February 3, 2016. https://blogs.uoregon.edu/richardtaylor/2016/02/03/human-physiological-responses-to-fractals-in-nature-and-art/.

Beresford-Kroeger, Diana. *Arboretum Borealis: A Lifeline of The Planet*. Ann Arbor: University of Michigan Press, 2010.

Beresford-Kroeger, Diana. *The Global Forest: 40 Ways Trees Can Save Us*. New York: Viking Penguin, 2010.

Beresford-Kroeger, Diana, Jeff McKay, Norman Dugas, Katsuhiko Matsunaga, and Akira Miyawaki. *Call of the Forest: The Forgotten Wisdom of Trees*. DVD. Directed by Jeff McKay. Winnipeg, Canada: Treespeak Films, 2016.

Berman, Marc, John Jonides, Stephen Kaplan. "The Cognitive Benefits of Interacting with Nature." *Psychological science* 19, no. 12 (2009): 1207–12. https://www.researchgate.com/publication/23718837_The_Cognitive_Benefits_of_Interacting_With_Nature/.

Bratman, Gregory N., Gretchen C. Daily, Benjamin J. Levy, James J. Gross. "The Benefits of Nature Experience: Improved Affect and Cognition." *Landscape and Urban Planning* 138 (2015): 41–50. https://www.sciencedirect.com/science/article/pii/S0169204615000286/.

Bratman, Gregory N., J. Paul Hamilton, Kevin S. Hahn, Gretchen C. Daily, and James J. Gross. "Nature Experience Reduces Rumination and Subgenual Prefrontal Cortex Activation." *Proceedings of the National Academy of Sciences* 112, no.28 (2015): 8567–8572. https://www.researchgate.net/publication/281315216_Nature_experience_reduces_rumination_and_subgenual_prefrontal_cortex_activation/.

Breedlove, Byron. "A Simple Sketch Symbolizing Self-Reliance." Emerging Infectious Diseases 22, no. 11 (2016): 2031–2032. https://www.ncbi.nlm.nih.gov/pmc/articles/PMC5088038/.

Brooks, Rebecca B. "The Life of Henry David Thoreau." *History of Massachusetts* (blog), February 20, 2017. https://historyofmassachusetts.org/henry-david-thoreau/.

Brown, Daniel K., Jo L. Barton, and Valerie F. Gladwell. "Viewing Nature Scenes Positively Affects Recovery of Autonomic Function Following Acute-Mental Stress." *Environmental Science & Technology* 47, no. 11 (2013): 5562–5569. https://www.ncbi.nlm.nih.gov/pubmed/23590163/.

Charles, Susan T., Jennifer R. Piazza, Jacqueline Mogle, Martin J. Sliwinski, David M. Almeida. "The Wear and Tear of Daily Stressors on Mental Health." *Psychological*

Science 24, no. 5 (2013): 733–741. https://doi.org/10.117 7%2F0956797612462222.

Crouse, Dan L., Lauren Pinault, Adele Balram, Perry Hystad, Paul A. Peters, Hong Chen, Aaron van Donkelaar, Randall V. Martin, Richard Ménard, Alain Robichaud, Paul J. Villeneuve. "Urban Greenness and Mortality in Canada's Largest Cities: A National Cohort Study." *The Lancet Planetary Health* 1, no 7 (2017): e289–e297. https://www.sciencedirect. com/science/article/pii/S2542519617301183/.

Crozier, Lorna. *The Wild in You: Voices from the Forest and the Sea*. Vancouver: Greystone Books, 2015.

Dillard, Annie. *The Writing Life*. New York: Harper Perennial, 1990.

Dockrill, Peter. "Doctors in Scotland Are Literally Prescribing Nature to Their Patients." *Science Alert*, October 9, 2018. https:// www.sciencealert.com/doctors-in-scotland-are-literally-pre-scribing-nature-to-patients-shetland-gps-pilot-benefits-health-mental/.

Falasinnu, Titilola, Yashaar Chaichian, and Julia F. Simard. "Impact of Sex on Systemic Lupus Erythematosus-Related Causes of Premature Mortality in the United States." Journal of Women's Health 26, no.1 (2017): 1214–1221. https://www. liebertpub.com/doi/full/10.1089/jwh.2017.6334/.

Fortier, Verla. "5 Reasons to Get Fit for the Outdoors." *Trees Mend Us* (blog). May 3, 2018. https://treesmendus. com/5-reasons-to-get-fit-for-the-outdoors/.

Fortier, Verla. "Break the Inside Habit (We Spend 93% of Our Time Inside)." *Trees Mend Us* (blog). May 10, 2018. https://treesmendus.com/ break-the-inside-habit-we-spend-93-of-our-time-inside/.

Fortier, Verla. "Health Benefits of Walking in the Trees with Poles." *Trees Mend Us* (blog). November 19, 2017. https:// treesmendus.com/health-benefits-of-trees-add-walking-poles/.

Gorman, James. "Finding Zen in a Patch of Nature." *The New York Times*. October 22, 2012. https://www.nytimes. com/2012/10/23/science/david-haskell-finds-biology-zen-in-a-patch-of-nature.html/.

Government of Canada. "Prevalence of Chronic Diseases Among Canadian Adults." Public Health Agency of Canada. Chronic Diseases. Last modified June 25, 2019. https://www.canada.ca/en/public-health/services/chronic-diseases/prevalence-canadian-adults-infographic-2019.html/.

Haskell, David G. *The Forest Unseen: A Year's Watch in Nature.* New York: Penguin Random House, 2013.

Haskell, David G. *The Songs of Trees: Stories From Nature's Great Connectors.* New York: Penguin Random House, 2018.

James, Peter, Jaime E. Hart, Rachel F. Banay, and Francine Ladena. "Exposure to Greenness and Mortality in a Nationwide Prospective Cohort Study of Women." *Environmental Health Perspectives* 124, no. 9 (2016). https://ehp.niehs.nih.gov/doi/10.1289/ehp.1510363/.

Jennifer R. Piazza, Susan T. Charles, Martin J. Sliwinski, Jacqueline Mogle J, David M. Almeida. "Affective Reactivity to Daily Stressors and Long-Term Risk of Reporting a Chronic Physical Health Condition." *Annals of Behavioral Medicine* 45, no. 1 (2013): 110–120. https://doi.org/10.1007/s12160-012-9423-0.

Juth, Vanessa, Joshua M. Smyth, Alecia M. Santuzzi. "How Do You Feel? Self-esteem Predicts Affect, Stress, Social Interaction, and Symptom Severity during Daily Life in Patients with Chronic Illness." Journal of Health Psychology 13, no. 7 (2008): 884–894. https://doi.org/10.1177%2F1359105308095062.

Kardan, Omid, Peter Gozdyra, Bratislav Misic, Faisal Moola, Lyle J. Palmer, Tomáš Paus, and Marc G. Berman, "Neighborhood green space and health in a large urban center," *Scientific Reports* 5, no. 11610 (2015). https://www.ncbi.nlm.nih.gov/pmc/articles/PMC4497305/.

Kimmerer, Robin W. *Gathering Moss: A Natural and Cultural History of Mosses.* Corvallis, OR: Oregon State University Press, 2017.

Klepeis, Neil E., William C. Nelson, Wayne R. Ott, John P. Robinson, Andy M. Tsang et.al. "The National Human Activity Pattern Survey (NHAPS): A Resource for Assessing Exposure to Environmental Pollutants." *Journal of Exposure Analysis and*

Environmental Epidemiology 11, (2001): 231–252. https://www.nature.com/articles/7500165#f1/.

Korpela, Kalevi, Matti Ylén, Liisa Tyrväinen, Harri Silvennoinen. "Favorite Green, Waterside and Urban Environments, Restorative Experiences and Perceived Health in Finland." *Health Promotion International* 25, no.2 (2010): 200–209. https://doi.org/10.1093/heapro/daq007.

Koyama, Alain, Jacqueline O'Brien, Jennifer Weuve, Deborah Blacker, Andrea L. Metti, Kristine Yaffe. The Role of Peripheral Inflammatory Markers in Dementia and Alzheimer's Disease: A Meta-Analysis." *The Journals of Gerontology: Series A* 68, no. 4 (2013): 433–440. https://doi.org/10.1093/gerona/gls187.

Kuhn, Simone, Sandra Düzel, Peter Eibich, Christian Krekel, Henry Wüstemann, Jens Kolbe, Johan Martensson, Jan Goebel, Jürgen Gallinat, Gert G. Wagner, and Ulman Lindenberger. "In Search of Features that Constitute an 'Enriched Environment' in Humans: Associations Between Geographical Properties and Brain Structure." *Scientific Reports* 7, no. 11920 (2017). https://www.nature.com/articles/s41598-017-12046-7/.

Lamott, Anne. *Bird by Bird: Some Instructions on Writing and Life*. New York: Pantheon Books, 1994.

Langer, Ellen J. *Mindfulness*. 25th Anniversary Edition. Philadephia: Da Capo Press, 2014.

Li, Qing. *Forest Bathing: How Trees Can Help You Find Health and Happiness.*New York: Viking Penguin, 2018.

Lovden, Martin, Elizabeth Wenger, Johan Martensson, Ulman Lindenberger, and Lars Backman. "Structural Brain Plasticity in Adult Learning and Development." *Neuroscience & Biobehavioral Reviews* 37, no. 9 (2013): 2296–2310. https://doi.org/10.1016/j.neubiorev.2013.02.014.

Lyubomirsky, Sonja, Kristin Layous, Joseph Chancellor, and S. Katherine Nelson. "Thinking About Rumination: The Scholarly Contributions and Intellectual Legacy of Susan Nolen-Hoeksema." Annual Review of Clinical Psychology 11, no.1 (2015): 1–22. https://www.annualreviews.org/doi/full/10.1146/annurev-clinpsy-032814-112733/.

Mayo Clinic. "Lupus." Patient Care & Health Information. Diseases & Conditions. October 25, 2017. https://www. mayoclinic.org/diseases-conditions/lupus/symptoms-causes/ syc-20365789/.

Neil, Kirsten. "Learning How to Care for Mother Earth." *CBC*, 2019. https://www.cbc.ca/news/canada/manitoba/events/ caring-for-mother-earth-1.5106422/.

Nisbet, Elizabeth, Melissa Lem. "Prescribing a Dose of Nature: Modern medicine is rediscovering the simple healing power of being outdoors." *Alternatives Journal*. Health 41.2 (2015). https://www.alternativesjournal.ca/sustainable-living/ prescribing-dose-nature/.

Nix, Steve. "A Beginner's Guide to Tree Identification." *ThoughtCo.* (blog), May 8, 2019. https://www.thoughtco.com/ identify-name-tree-using-leaf-key-1343488/.

Nix, Steve. "What Is Diameter Breast Height? One of the Most Important Tree Measurements for Foresters." *ThoughtCo.* (blog), March 7, 2019. https://www.thoughtco.com/ what-is-diameter-breast-height-1341720/.

Nolen-Hoeksema, Susan. *Eating, Drinking, and Over-thinking*. New York: Henry Holt and Company, LLC, 2006.

Nolen-Hoeksema, Susan. *Women Who Think Too Much: How to Break Free of Overthinking and Reclaim Your Life*. New York: Henry Holt and Company, LLC, 2004.

Nordixx. "International Overview on Clinical & Scientific Studies on Nordic Pole Walking General Studies." Scientific Studies. https://www.nordixx.com/pages/scientific-studies/.

Nutt, Kristy. "Nature to Be Prescribed to Help Health and Wellbeing." *The Royal Society for the Protection of Birds*, October 5, 2018. https://www.rspb.org.uk/ about-the-rspb/about-us/media-centre/press-releases/ nature-prescribed-to-help-health/#FJiSPDXgeBg891lm.99/.

O'Donnell, Ellen. "Bratman Describes Science of Nature's Effects on Psychological Health." National Institutes of Health LXX, no. 25 (2018). https://nihrecord.nih.gov/newslet-ters/2018/12_14_2018/story4.htm/.

Park, Bum Jin, Yuko Tsunetsugu, Tamami Kasetani, Takahide Kagawa, and Yoshifumi Miyazaki. "The physiological effects of Shinrin-yoku (taking in the forest atmosphere or forest bathing): evidence from field experiments in 24 forests across Japan." *Environmental Health and Preventive Medicine* 15 (2010): 18–26. https://doi.org/10.1007/s12199-009-0086-9.

Parsons, Russ, Louis G. Tassinary, Roger S. Ulrich, Michelle R. Hebl, Michele Grossman-Alexander. "The View from the Road: Implications for Stress Recovery and Immunization." *Journal of Environmental Psychology* 18, no 2 (1998): 113–140. https://doi.org/10.1006/jevp.1998.0086.

Penn, Joanna. *How to Write Non-Fiction: Turn Your Knowledge into Words (Books for Writers)*. Bath, UK: Curl Up Press, 2018.

Piff, Paul K., Pia Dietze, Matthew Feinberg, Daniel M. Stancato, Dacher Keltner. "Awe, the Small Self, and prosocial Behavior." *Journal of Personality and Social Psychology* 108, no. 6 (2015): 883-899. http://doi.org/10.1037/pspi0000018.

Pinto, Yair, Andries R. van der Leij, Ilja G. Sligte, Victor A. F. Lamme, H. Steven Scholte. "Bottom-Up and Top-Down Attention Are Independent," Journal of Vision 13, no.3 (2013). https://jov.arvojournals.org/article.aspx?articleid=2194099/.

Plassman, Brenda L, Kenneth M. Langa, Ryan J. McCammon, Gwenith G. Fisher, Guy G. Potter, James R. Burke, et al. "Incidence of Dementia and Cognitive Impairment, Not Dementia in the United States." *Annals of Neurology* 70, no. 3 (2011): 418–426. https://doi.org/10.1002/ana.22362.

Ramsayer, Kate. "Help NASA Measure Trees with Your Smartphone." *NASA*. March 26, 2019. https://www.nasa.gov/feature/goddard/2019/help-nasa-measure-trees-with-new-app/.

Sawatsky, Jarem. *Dancing with Elephants*. Winnipeg, Canada: Red Canoe Press, 2017.

Scott, Stacey B., Jennifer E. Graham-Engeland, Christopher G. Engeland, Joshua M. Smyth, David M. Almeida, Mindy J. Katz, Richard B. Lipton, Jacqueline A. Mogle, Elizabeth Munoz, Nilam Ram, and Martin J. Sliwinski. "The Effects of Stress on Cognitive Aging, Physiology and Emotion (ESCAPE) Project."

BMC Psychiatry 15, no. 146 (2015). https://doi.org/10.1186/s12888-015-0497-7.

Takayama, Norimasa, Kalevi Korpela, Juyoung Lee, Takeshi Morikawa, Yuko Tsunetsugu, Bum-Jin Park, Qing Li et.al. "Emotional, Restorative and Vitalizing Effects of Forest and Urban Environments at Four Sites in Japan." International Journal of Environmental Research and Public Health 11, no. 7 (2014): 7207-7230. https://doi.org/10.3390/ijerph110707207.

Taylor, Richard P., and Branka Spehar. "Fractal Fluency: An Intimate Relationship Between the Brain and Processing of Fractal Stimuli." In *The Fractal Geometry of the Brain*, edited by Antonio Di Ieva, 485–496. New York: Springer-Verlag, 2016.

The Fractal Foundation. "What Is a Fractal." Index of Fractivities. August 18, 2009. https://fractalfoundation.org/fractivities/WhatIsaFractal-1pager.pdf/.

Thoreau, Henry David. "Walking." *The Atlantic*. June 1862. https://www.theatlantic.com/magazine/archive/1862/06/walking/304674/.

Tinker, Ann. "How to Improve Patient Outcomes for Chronic Diseases and Comorbidities." *Health Catalyst*, 2017. https://www.healthcatalyst.com/wp-content/uploads/2014/04/How-to-Improve-Patient-Outcomes.pdf/.

Tippett, Krista. "Ellen Langer: Science of Mindlessness and Mindfulness." *On Being with Krista Tippett* (blog). Last Updated November 2, 2017. https://onbeing.org/programs/ellen-langer-science-of-mindlessness-and-mindfulness-nov2017/.

Tippett, Krista. "Robin Wall Kimmerer: The Intelligence in All Kinds of Life." *On Being with Krista Tippett* (blog). Last Updated July 19, 2018. https://onbeing.org/programs/robin-wall-kimmerer-the-intelligence-in-all-kinds-of-life-jul2018/.

Trent University. "Your Happiness Could Depend on the Time You Spend Outdoors." News and Events. https://www.trentu.ca/news/story/15885?&newsId=15885/.

Ulrich R.S. "View through a window may influence recovery from surgery." *Science* 224, no. 4647 (1984): 420–421. https://science.sciencemag.org/content/224/4647/420/.

Ulrich R.S., R.F. Simons, B.D. Losito, E. Fiorito, M.A. Miles, M. Zelson. "Stress Recovery During Exposure to Natural and Urban Environments." *Journal of Environmental Psychology* 11, no. 3 (1991): 201–230. https://doi.org/10.1016/S0272-4944(05)80184-7.

University of Minnesota. "Let's Talk about Mindfulness: An Interview with Ellen Langer." *Taking Charge of Your Health & Wellbeing* video, 11:21. November 24, 2014. https://www.takingcharge.csh.umn.edu/lets-talk-about-mindfulness-interview-ellen-langer/.

Van den Berg, Agnes E., Jolanda Maas, Robert A. Verheij, Peter P. Groenewegen. "Green Space as a Buffer Between Stressful Life Events and Health." *Social Science & Medicine* 70, no. 8 (2010): 1203–121. https://www.sciencedirect.com/science/article/abs/pii/S0277953610000675?via%3Dihub/.

Van den Berg, Magdalena M.H.E., Jolanda Maas, Rianne Muller, Anoek Braun, Wendy Kaandorp, René Van Lien, Mireille N.M. Van Poppel, Willem Van Mechelen, and Agnes E. Van den Berg. "Autonomic Nervous System Responses to Viewing Green and Built Settings: Differentiating Between Sympathetic and Parasympathetic Activity." *International Journal of Environmental Research and Public Health* 12, no.12 (2015): 15860–15874. https://doi.org/10.3390/ijerph121215026.

Wichmann, Margarete A., Karen J. Cruickshanks, Cynthia M. Carlsson, Rick Chappell, Mary E. Fischer, Barbara E. K. Klein, Ronald Klein, et al. "Long-Term Systemic Inflammation and Cognitive Impairment in a Population-Based Cohort." *Journal of the American Geriatrics Society* 62, no. 9 (2014): 1683–1691. https://doi.org/10.1111/jgs.12994.

Williams, Florence. *The Nature Fix: Why Nature Makes Us Happier, Healthier, and More Creative.* New York: W.W. Norton & Company Ltd, 2017.

Wilson, Robert S., David A. Bennett, Carlos F. Mendes de Leon, Julia L. Bienias, Martha C. Morris, Denis A. Evans. "Distress Proneness and Cognitive Decline in a Population of Older Persons." *Psychoneuroendocrinology* 30, no. 1 (2005): 11–17. https://doi.org/10.1016/j.psyneuen.2004.04.005.

Printed in Great Britain
by Amazon